WHEN YOU HAVE CHEST PAINS

OTHER BOOKS BY
GERSHON LESSER:

Growing Younger: Nutritional Rejuvenation for People over Forty

Lowell House
Los Angeles

Contemporary Books
Chicago

WHEN YOU HAVE CHEST PAINS

A Guide to
Cardiac and Noncardiac Causes
and What You Can Do About Them

GERSHON LESSER, M.D.
LARRY STRAUSS

Copyright © 1989 by RGA Publishing Group, Inc.

All rights reserved. No part of this work may be reproduced or transmitted in any form or by any means, electronic or mechanical, including photocopying and recording, or by any information storage or retrieval system, except as may be expressly permitted by the 1976 Copyright Act or in writing by the publisher.
Requests for such permission should be addressed to:

Lowell House
1950 Sawtelle Blvd.
Los Angeles, CA 90025

Library of Congress Cataloging-in-Publication Data

Lesser, Gershon M.
  When you have chest pains.

  Bibliography: p.
  Includes index.
  1. Chest pain—Popular works. 2. Coronary heart diseases—Diagnosis—Popular works. 3. Diagnosis, Differential. I. Strauss, Larry. II. Title.
RC941.L49   1989   617'.5407'5   89-2440
ISBN 0-929923-02-2

Design: Barbara Monahan
Manufactured in the United States of America
10 9 8 7 6 5 4 3 2 1

To
Michelle, Hadrian, Aaron, and Jason,
and Mom

—GERSHON M. LESSER, M.D.

To
Mom and Dad

—LARRY STRAUSS

CONTENTS

Acknowledgments   xi
A Cautionary Note   xiii
Introduction:
If You Can't Prevent a Heart Attack,
You Might As Well Survive It   1

PART ONE: NONCARDIAC CAUSES OF CHEST PAIN   9

Esophageal-Related Chest Pain   12
Stomach-Related Chest Pain   29
Pancreas-Related Chest Pain   40
Gallbladder-Related Chest Pain   43
Pulmonary-Related Chest Pain   46
Mediastinal Chest Pain   67
Chest Wall Pain   72
Other Physical Noncardiac Conditions Known to Cause Chest Pain   79
Psychological Causes of Chest Pain   85

PART TWO: WHEN YOUR HEART SPEAKS, LISTEN!   95

  Angina   99

  Heart Irregularity   114

  Pericarditis   119

  Myocarditis   122

  Syphilitic Heart Disease   125

  Left Ventricular Hypertrophy   128

  Valve Disorders   131

  Bacterial Endocarditis   136

  Cardiomyopathy   137

  Cardiac Tumors   139

  Heart Attack   140

PART THREE: ANSWERING PAIN WITH ACTION   149

  Preparation for and Relaxation During the Most Stressful Moments of Your Life   151

  The Fifty-Year Cholesterol and Hypertension Plan   168

Beyond Latin: The Glossary 211
Resources 217
Recommended Reading 219
Index 221

ACKNOWLEDGMENTS

We wish to express our gratitude to Jack Artenstein, who had the vision to publish a book about the ever-important issue of chest pain, and to Janice Gallagher, whose editorial vigor helped to shape this book.

We would also like to express thanks to the many people whose encouragement and wisdom have helped to inspire us: Dr. Linus Pauling, Dr. Albert Zager, Dr. James D. Boyle, Dr. Gerald Federman, Dr. George Griffith, Dr. Thomas Brem, Dr. Peter Gabor, Dr. Lewis Cozen, Dr. Mark Tobenkin, Dr. Ernie Shore, Dr. James Kleinenberg, Dr. Myron Rosenbaum, Dr. Donald Rossman, Dr. Elliot Blinderman, Dr. Joseph Schachtman, Dr. Jerome Tamkin, David Zeitlin of the Los Angeles County Medical Association, Jeff Cory, Norma Barzman, Ellis St. Joseph, Michael Barb, Ruth Hirschman, Will Lewis, Mitchell Harding, Robert Forst, Dick McGeary, Mike Lundy, Ray Breim, Geoff Edwards, George Kostka, Jim Simon, John Swaney, Bill Barry, the wonderful people of A.M. Northwest in Portland, Irv Atkins, Max Candiotty, David Dutton, Irwin Zucker, Carole Schild, Commander and Mrs. Robert Manheim and the Rotarians of Greater Los Angeles, Steven Knight, James A. Stearn, Dr. Earl Mindell, Dr. Joyce Shulman and Dr. Lee Shulman, and all the loyal and loving patients along with the many *Health Connection* listeners everywhere.

A CAUTIONARY NOTE

The nature of medical practice and information is flux and change, not the stability some of us may like to believe exists. More so than in almost any other science, facts and beliefs in medicine have the characteristic of never standing still. What we believe today we must be prepared to alter or discard tomorrow based on new observations. While in the past it took decades, even centuries, to revise such standardized practices as the use of leeches and ether, today new insights occur with the speed of light; the half-life of a medical fact in the twentieth century is about one week.

I urge you, therefore, not to use this book as a substitute for the advice of your competent physician and counselor. My purpose in writing it is not to suggest that all is known —about chest pain or any other medical issue—or that what applies to one person applies collectively to everyone. Nor do I, herewith, offer prescriptions or medical cures. What's good for me may be harmful for you, and vice versa. No book can know an individual as well as a physician's listening ear and searching eye. Furthermore, reasonable argument can probably present a case opposite to every suggestion made in this or any other book regarding the prevention, cause, symptoms, and treatment of any illness. No recommendation, after all, comes without some potential for risk. Even aspirin, we now know, can cause lethal hemorrhages and ulcers in some people.

In every case, symptoms represent significant body messages. Some are benign and need simple responses. Some are potentially messages of serious, even lethal, conditions. A pain always requires an explanation, and a trained physician should be sought out to this end. Even the immediate response of a paramedic may be the only reasonable action you must take. It is folly to ignore your chest pain. But knowledge concerning the various kinds and causes will give you the calm and the control to deal with them in an orderly and unfearful manner.

I offer my observations not as the "final word" in any sense, but as a starting point in the process of personal growth and the kind of awareness that can enhance your life.

GERSHON M. LESSER, M.D.

INTRODUCTION: IF YOU CAN'T PREVENT A HEART ATTACK, YOU MIGHT AS WELL SURVIVE IT

I hope that you never have a heart attack. I also hope that you are never caught in an earthquake, a hurricane, a flood, or a fire. Statistically, that is impossible. I may be an outspoken practitioner of preventive medicine and, yes, I've said many times that heart disease is, in the vast majority of cases, a choice and not an inevitability of genetics—but I am also a realist. Even today, with the tremendous awareness about the containment of heart disease through diet and lifestyle modifications, heart attacks happen. They happen to my friends as well as yours. In Los Angeles, where I live, we are urged constantly by public service messages to prepare our homes and families for that impending 8.9 on the Richter scale. Earthquake survival guides are handed out at parades and sent free of charge in the mail, informing us how much food and water and cash to stockpile, where to stand during a tremor and its aftershocks. Yet no earthquake could ever threaten so many lives as heart attacks do every year.

According to the American Heart Association (AHA), one and a half million people will suffer a heart attack during the next twelve months. But only about a third of these heart attacks will be fatal. Having a heart attack does not mean you are going to die. Thanks in part to modern medicine and in part to the endurance of the human body and the resilience of the human spirit, millions of people, including many of my own friends and patients, have rebounded from a coronary thrombosis, often with a new attitude toward life and tremendous potential for good health and longevity. "So you weren't able to prevent a heart attack," I tell those of my patients, with a shrug. "Thank God you survived it."

Let this be *your* survival guide.

The information in these pages will prepare you not only to survive that heart attack I hope you *never* have but also will enable you to help your husband or wife or mother or father—or whomever—survive the heart attack I hope *they* never have. Taking the time to read this book is a kind of insurance policy; it is also an act of love.

There is no physical symptom more frightening than a chest pain. Discovering blood in our urine or a growth on the neck or breast may be terrifying, but they do not threaten instant mortality. Well, neither should a chest pain, not if we want to maximize our chances of survival. We need to respect the danger we are in and its immediacy, and we need to act fast, but we also need to think clearly and to be calm. A little knowledge can help immeasurably. When the topic is chest pain, ignorance is *not* bliss.

In addition to being the most frightening of all symptoms, chest pain is also among the most common. In my own practice, it is rare when a week goes by that I have not seen 10 to 15 patients with chest pain. About one in every four patients pays me a visit because of a chest pain. And, strange as it may seem, I sometimes wish I had twice as many, because probably half of all sufferers of chest pain choose to confront the problem not with medical diagnosis and intervention but with denial.

This, I have discovered, is a tragedy of major proportions. Every year half a million people die of a heart attack. Most begin with a chest pain and many, if dealt with immediately, could have been treated—as in the case of the more than one million people who *survive* heart attacks each year. No one is certain why chest pain denial is so widespread (or why, ironically, physicians themselves are the single largest group of chest pain denial victims), but I believe that the knowledge presented in these pages can help to combat this game of anatomical Russian roulette by offering a respect for the various causes of chest pain along with an understanding that, in most cases, the danger increases exponentially with the delay of denial. The difference between acceptance and denial can be the difference between full recuperation and permanent cardiac damage; it can be the difference between survival and death. We have all heard stories of someone found dead of heart failure with a roll of antacid just below his or her limp hand. We have also heard about the countless men and women rushed through the doors of emergency wards clutching their breastbones only to discover that what they are suffering from is too much chili. Some of them might feel pretty foolish, mistaking heartburn for a heart attack. They are not foolish. Foolish is dying on your mattress, trying to treat a coronary with bicarbonate.

There are many possible causes for chest pain: some minor, some serious, some (not just cardiac in nature) life-threatening. All must be considered life-threatening until diagnosed otherwise. The severity of the pain has no direct correlation to the seriousness of its cause. Emotionally induced chest pain, for example, can be unimaginably excruciating; yet, in and of itself, it presents no *immediate* danger. The pain of a coronary may not be incapacitating—until it is too late.

A few years ago a 48-year-old colleague of mine was in the midst of hosting a dinner party when he felt a mild pain in his upper torso. He mentioned it to his wife and asked her for some Pepto-Bismol. His wife asked, "If you're having a chest pain, shouldn't we have it checked out at the emergency room?" My colleague, God bless him, responded with,

"Now, honey, that's being awfully neurotic, isn't it?" And, with that, he marched into the bathroom and helped himself to the renowned pink medicine.

His wife kept a close eye on him and saw that he remained in discomfort. About an hour later when their guests had departed, she insisted they go get him an electrocardiogram (EKG). My colleague insisted that he felt fine but didn't feel like arguing; so, he complied. When they reached the hospital, he no longer felt fine. In the middle of the EKG began the acute pain of a coronary.

Talk about being in the right place at the right time. Within minutes he was on the operating table, a blood clot was located and dissolved, and he was fully recovered. Not one cell of his heart tissue sustained any damage. Had his wife listened to him—had she not persisted in her concern—he ran all the risks of suffering an acute coronary, including ventricular fibrillation, cardiac standstill, and death before the paramedics might even have arrived. Even if the ambulance had arrived in time, all the heart tissue beyond the clotted blood vessel would likely have been dead tissue, leaving him at significant risk for future cardiac illness.

How you choose to react to a chest pain could be one of the most—if not *the* most—important decisions you will ever make. It is, therefore, a decision that should be made long before you ever *have* a chest pain. It is a decision I urge you to make right now. A recent, rather disturbing, study in the *Internal Medicine News* found that an alarming number of cardiac patients leave emergency rooms against the advice of the staff cardiologist and found that in the vast majority of cases these people are *not* as well as they believe they are.

Do not play doctor with your chest pain—or with anyone else's. As zealous as I may feel about quality health being the patient's responsibility, self-diagnosis of a chest pain is a skydive with an untested parachute.

Do not use this book as a tool for self-diagnosis.

Not just because you might die of a heart attack. The

potential of a coronary is not the only reason to take chest pain seriously. Chest pain can be a symptom of many other serious conditions, such as esophageal disorder, chest wall disorder, skeletal abnormality, disc syndrome, muscle disease, tumor, pulmonary hypertension, infection, virus, pancreatic or gallbladder disease, chronic fatigue, duodenal ulcer, high blood pressure, depression, and panic attack, as well as noncoronary heart problems such as cardiac inflammation and dissecting aortic aneurism. All of these conditions are addressed in the sections contained in Part One of the book, *Noncardiac Causes of Chest Pain*. Part Two, *When Your Heart Speaks, Listen!*, deals with the cardiac causes of chest pain.

Virtually every chest pain is a potentially serious matter. Even if it does *not* pose any immediate peril, many of these illnesses, over time, can increase greatly the risk of heart attack; so, dealing with the problem now by *responding to a doctor's diagnosis and treatment* can serve as an effective preventive measure.

No, I cannot save you any potentially unnecessary calls to the paramedics or trips to the emergency room. To do so would be to encourage you to unnecessarily risk your health and your life. What I can do is suggest ways in which you can reduce the chances of having heartburn or of allowing unresolved emotional stresses to induce chest pain. More important, I will in Part Three, *Answering Pain with Action*, suggest ways to increase your chances not only of surviving a heart attack but also of surviving any chest pain emergency, including ways to control stress during what may very well be the most stressful moments of your life. Following *Preparation For and Relaxation During the Most Stressful Moments of Your Life* is *The 50-Year Cholesterol and Hypertension Plan*, in which I suggest how, on a more than temporary basis, you can reduce greatly the risk of ever having a heart attack or other cardiac chest pain emergency. In fact, this information—some of which you may already know but choose to ignore, some you may have forgotten, and some of which you may not have heard—can promote not only a healthy cardiovascular system but also general overall health and thus may reduce the risk of noncardiac chest pain emergencies as well.

Sometimes half the battle in maintaining health and ensuring longevity is won through gaining a basic understanding of how your body works and doesn't work and what enhances health and what does not. I am an advocate of clear and simple communication between doctor and patient, and so I will try to avoid flaunting my Latin vocabulary at you. There are, however, some terms that it is important to use and to define for you (in case your life is ever in the hands of a doctor who does *not* try to avoid flaunting his or her Latin vocabulary at you). I will define all such medical terminology first in the text and again in the glossary.

Actually, when I say "I," I mean "we" (we mean "we") —this being the composite voice of Gershon Lesser, M.D., and Larry Strauss—which brings us to the format of this book: question and answer.

Dr. Lesser, an internist and cardiologist for over 20 years and a medical journalist for over 10, has come to regard listening to his patients and his radio listeners and answering their questions as essential ingredients of effective medicine. Strauss, a long-time listener and patient of Dr. Lesser, is well aware of just how crucial it is to ask any doctor the right questions. Such as:

What if I have a chest pain at four o'clock in the morning? Do I have to get out of bed, get dressed, and drive to the hospital?

You can have a heart attack at any time, day or night. It doesn't matter if you've had a hundred chest pains before that turned out to be nothing. Don't let that give you a false sense of security. And I wouldn't recommend driving yourself to the hospital when you are having a chest pain. Call the paramedics.

What if I'm 22 years old and have no personal or genetic history of heart disease?

Many chest pain causes are totally unexpected and are not age-related.

But if it's not a coronary, I'm not going to die if I wait until 7 A.M., right?

Wrong. I wouldn't take the chance—nor would I let you take that chance. The problem could be in the lungs or in the lining of the lungs or heart. You could be bleeding internally. Time is of the essence.

What if the pain goes away before I get my pants on?

That depends on how long it takes you to get your pants on. If the pain occurs for only an instant and if you have no reason to suspect it might indicate a serious condition, you could wait, paying close attention for any recurrence. However, if a chest pain persists for more than a few minutes, call the paramedics. Or call your doctor and let him or her call the paramedics. If you don't have a doctor and the paramedics are on strike or you live in a place without paramedics, have someone drive you to the nearest emergency room.

What if the pain subsides to the point where I can easily fall back to sleep? I mean, if it's serious, it would keep me awake, right?

You really don't want to get out of that bed, do you? Unfortunately, although the fervor of denial can overcome pain with remarkable adroitness, you *cannot* will yourself out of a coronary or a hemorrhagic pericardial effusion or a fractured rib or a pulmonary blood clot or any of the other serious causes of chest pain.

Part One
NONCARDIAC CAUSES OF CHEST PAIN

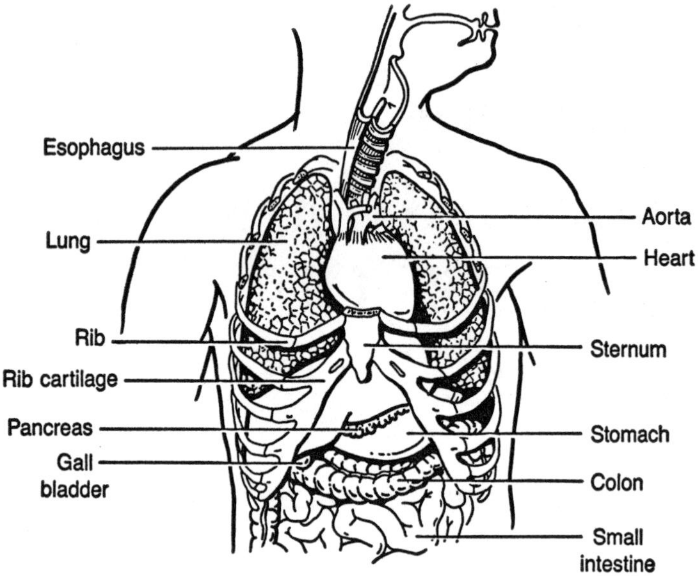
Esophagus
Aorta
Lung
Heart
Rib
Sternum
Rib cartilage
Pancreas
Stomach
Gall bladder
Colon
Small intestine

FIGURE 1

Looking at figure 1, you can see that the cardiac neighborhood is quite crowded. This is, of course, out of necessity. Lungs flank the heart in order to keep up with its enormous oxygen demands. The stomach sits at an easily accessible distance to make its contribution. The esophagus passes parallel to the heart, this being the shortest route from mouth to stomach. The skeleton encases the heart and its neighbors protectively; the spinal cord and column with all its muscles sit inches away. Think of the heart as the centerpiece of the human organ puzzle and it is not difficult to imagine why noncardiac chest pain is so common.

Esophageal-Related Chest Pain

What is an esophagus and what does mine do for me?

The esophagus is the tube-like muscle connecting the mouth and throat to the stomach. Its purpose is to allow food to make its downward journey and to allow gas and, if necessary, vomit to flow out of the stomach.

And what is the most common kind of esophageal chest pain?

Heartburn—clinically known as *reflux esophagitis* (heartburn) or, more specifically, *gastroesophageal reflux* (burning of the esophagus by hydrochloric acid from the stomach).

So, heartburn has nothing to do with the heart?

Nothing whatsoever. Heartburn happens when not-yet-fully-digested food, saturated with stomach acid, gets flung from the stomach back up into the esophagus. The stomach acid burns the delicate lining of the esophagus.

Why would my stomach want to fling undigested food up into my esophagus?

It doesn't want to. In fact, in most cases, the stomach is not the culprit. A very common cause of heartburn is the result of a weak or malfunctioning sphincter muscle at the base of the esophagus. Sphincter muscles—of which we have several throughout our bodies—are designed to close tightly and then open upon necessity. The sphincter you would be most aware of is your anus. Most of the time it remains closed so tightly that you can take a bath or jump into a pool without the slightest worry that water will surge up your rectum. Yet when nature calls, it relaxes accordingly. The sphincter at the base of the esophagus works in much the same way —when it works. It relaxes to allow the downward flow of food into the stomach. Then, once all of the food has flowed into the stomach, this sphincter shuts tightly so that the stomach can begin secreting hydrochloric acid and churning in its digestive process. Think of it this way: If the door of a clothing dryer fails to remain closed during its spin, something is likely to fly out.

When I get heartburn, all I'm feeling is stomach acid on my esophagus?

Hydrochloric acid (HCl) is among the most powerful acids. You could burn a hole in the side of your house with HCl. Fortunately, your stomach comes equipped with a protective mucous lining that is impervious to this incendiary acid. Because it is designed to transport food *before* it becomes saturated with HCl, your esophagus does not. When stomach acid splatters against the walls of your esophagus, the pain can be excruciating. It is usually *substernal* (below the breastbone), sharp, and intense. To anyone who has had a coronary, this pain can feel frighteningly similar; to anyone who has *not* had a coronary, it can feel exactly as he or she might imagine one.

14 NONCARDIAC CAUSES OF CHEST PAIN

Why would the sphincter muscle at the base of my esophagus want to put me through all this?

There are a number of possible reasons for that muscle not to be doing its job correctly, but the most common cause happens to be chocolate. A chemical in chocolate can cause this sphincter muscle to relax when it is supposed to contract. People with reflux esophagitis are often told not to eat chocolate. Excessive alcohol consumption can also instigate the same sphincter relaxation in many people. The third chemical culprit is caffeine. After that, the list of offenders would probably include excess refined sugars and carbohydrates, followed by excess saturated fats. Sphincter relaxation can also be symptomatic of *any* food allergy. It can also be a side effect of many different medications, both over-the-counter and prescription. Over-the-counter deep-sleep medications, for example, are designed to relax the body and mind; in many people they also relax the sphincter muscle we've been talking about, causing heartburn (and very likely ruining the deep sleep that the user is seeking). Antihistamines, which have a relaxing action on some muscles, may also produce this side effect. Very common prescription medicines known to cause reflux esophagitis include estrogen and progesterone—commonly taken by women to treat menopausal symptoms.

It can also be caused by another physical illness known as hiatal hernia, which is a sliding of the stomach upward through the diaphragm and into the chest alongside the esophagus—where it most certainly does not belong.

What about jalapeño peppers and hot Chinese mustard?

There is no question that spicy foods can cause a burning of the esophagus wall—and the pain called heartburn. But usually, if these foods are eaten in moderation, the burning will only occur in those people for whom spicy foods stimulate excess stomach acid secretion or cause the relaxation of the sphincter muscle or whose esophagus lining is already injured from recurring bouts with reflux esophagitis. In the latter case, the pain would be felt while eating.

A much more likely cause for heartburn occurs when these foods—or any foods for that matter—are *over*eaten. Overeating is a very common cause of reflux esophagitis. Let's face it, if you heap too much food into the confines of your stomach, once it starts churning, your sphincter muscle —even if it's in great shape—isn't going to be able to contain the tidal wave of your excesses; in fact, if you fill your stomach and continue eating, the sphincter has no choice but to remain open, regardless of whether digestion has begun.

Why do pregnant women frequently complain of heartburn?

As the womb and its fetus grow, they decrease the capacity of the abdomen and exert pressure upon surrounding tissues and organs. What was once a moderate amount of food now overloads the stomach, and the result is the same as when a nonpregnant person overeats. Pregnancy is, of course, a temporary condition. Once the stomach is able to reclaim its turf within the abdomen, the pregnancy-related heartburn problem should subside before any long-term damage to the esophagus is sustained. However, since the discomfort can make for an unpleasant pregnancy, I usually recommend eating many very small meals to avoid overloading the stomach at any given time.

What if my heartburn is not caused by pregnancy? What do I do about it?

First you have to determine that it *is* heartburn. Only a doctor can make that diagnosis. Then you need to eliminate —or greatly reduce the consumption of—all foods and other substances most likely to be the culprit. Since many of these substances are health hazards, to some degree, I would not consider such a measure impetuous. For good measure, let's recap the list of substances known to cause reflux esophagitis in some people:

Chocolate; alcohol (including beer and wine); caffeine (and that includes many over-the-counter medications); refined sugars and carbohydrates; saturated fats; cigarettes; any over-the-counter deep-sleep, wake-up, or so-called diet pills; and antihistamines.

Your doctor would probably also recommend avoiding foods that increase acid production: milk and other dairy products, doughnuts, even potentially vitamin C, as well as chocolate, alcohol, and coffee—all of which we are already avoiding because of their effect on sphincter relaxation.

It is probably also a good idea to go easy on foods that are themselves high in acid: vinegar, citrus fruits, spices, hot peppers, horseradish, and any fermented product.

I would also advise you to avoid or greatly reduce consumption of soda pop and other carbonated beverages; the phosphoric acid has been known to cause a burning of the esophagus lining in some people. Of course, use common sense and avoid any particular foods experience has shown to cause you heartburn. And, *stop overeating.* Also avoid lying down right after *any* size meal—use gravity to *help* digestion flow painlessly.

If the problem of heartburn persists and the pain becomes excruciating, your doctor will likely prescribe Tagamet, Zantac, Pepcid, or anticholinergic, such as Bentyl. Anticholinergic is the fancy name for a kind of medicine that reduces acid production in the stomach. These medications can be effective in the treatment of gastritis but there can be side effects. Tagamet (a.k.a. cimetidine) has been found, in a few cases, to cause impotence, and, in combination with some other drugs, mental confusion, and even breast growth in males. It may also reduce the effectiveness of some other medications, such as blood thinners, asthma drugs, some blood pressure drugs, and even such tranquilizers as Valium. Fortunately, most of these side effects can be reversed by replacing Tagamet with another medicine.

Beware of painkillers when dealing with chest pain of any kind. After all, you wouldn't want to get into the habit of suppressing a feeling that might, one day, save your life. I'm not suggesting you should endure an excruciating pain —as long as you are just as zealous about working with your doctor to diagnose and treat its cause. If the cause of your heartburn is the result of overeating or some other behavior, why not simply let the pain motivate the termination of that behavior?

Some simple and sometimes effective remedies for the pain of heartburn include drinking cold water, which can be the *most* effective remedy. One to two glasses of H_2O may be all that is needed to cool off the esophagus lining and ease the pain. Elevating the head during sleep (keeping it at a higher level than the stomach) may help prevent those 4 A.M. heartburn attacks.

What about antacids?

I purposely avoided mentioning antacids earlier because I deplore them as among the most overused over-the-counter drugs (OTCs) on the market. Since you asked, antacids are supposed to neutralize the excess acid in the esophagus (or stomach). Remember in junior high school when your science teacher made you dip litmus paper into different solutions to determine whether they were acids or bases? Then he or she probably explained that acids neutralize bases and vice versa. The neutralization process transforms the acid into water and a salt. Sometimes antacids work, sometimes they don't. Their efficacy probably depends upon the amount of acid causing the discomfort, since the strength of the antacid base is a constant. Antacids, at best, treat only the painful symptoms, not the underlying long-term effects of the constant singeing of the inner walls of the esophagus by the acid.

And there are a number of potential side effects. Regular use of these products can cause acid rebound, making heartburn even worse. Regular use can also block the body's absorption of iron and vitamin B_{12}, which eventually can lead to anemia. Also, some antacids are high in aluminum, which can compromise the body's ability to absorb calcium, increasing the long-term risk of osteoporosis and other bone disease. Excess aluminum in the brain has been linked to a greater risk of Alzheimer's disease. Some antacids are high in sodium, increasing the risk of high blood pressure. Regular use of antacids has been responsible, in some people, for reducing the ability to taste.

I'm afraid to ask about the long-term effects of perennial heartburn.

Now that you've brought it up, the constant assault on the inside of the esophagus can cause its erosion. Mild bleeding and an unexplained iron-deficiency anemia may ensue. An eroded esophagus is a common cause of recurring laryngitis. Esophageal erosion can also lead to a disease called Barrett's esophagus, in which the cells in the esophagus wall stop producing mucus and become nonelastic. If not treated, these cells will eventually become cancerous. Reflux esophagitis can be accompanied by lung infection if the reflux of HCl and other stomach contents reaches the lung.

Would I have any way of knowing whether heartburn had caused any of these illnesses?

The only way to know for certain is from a doctor's diagnosis. Because a well-informed patient is almost always a better patient and because this kind of knowledge might motivate someone not to let his or her heartburn lead to other illnesses, here goes.

Esophageal erosion is characterized by frequent heartburn and recurring chest pain that is substernal and constant and that seems to occur at rest or when not eating or digesting food. Other symptoms are progressively painful swallowing, bloody vomit, black, tar-like stool, and, all too often, unnoticeable internal bleeding. It is usually diagnosed with X rays or scopes.

Barrett's esophagus usually causes painful swallowing and chest pain and often causes food to get stuck in the esophagus. A biopsy is usually needed to make this diagnosis.

Cancer of the esophagus can cause any of the symptoms previously mentioned—or no symptoms at all. Sometimes there is weight loss. Biopsy is the diagnostic tool for this cancer.

Lung infections are often the cause of recurring cough, thick and/or colored sputum, fever, chills, debility, shortness of breath, and sweating. Diagnosis can be made with X rays, scopes, and cultures.

Having said all that, I must further state it has been my experience that the most likely danger of untreated—or unprevented—heartburn is that it can cause complacency with regard to chest pain. You might begin to take it for granted: "It's just my old friend, heartburn." And you never really know if it is. Such a false sense of security can be life-threatening. I'm not just talking about a heart attack either. I'm also talking about noncardiac causes of chest pain. There are other esophageal disorders—often mistaken for heartburn—which can, if not treated, be life-threatening.

And these have nothing to do with stomach acid or sphincter muscles?

Stomach acid is not the problem, but sphincter muscles are. There is another of these tightly wound apertures at the other end of the esophagus which, when it is functioning normally, relaxes during food or liquid consumption, then tightens during digestion so that no reflux splashes into the back of the throat or the mouth. It is also designed to relax at the upward flow of gas, which allows us to belch. The problem arises when this reflex fails—the upper sphincter fails to open—and the gas gets stuck in the esophagus.

Why does this sphincter fail to open?

The cause is still controversial—which means as of this writing there is no generally accepted theory.

And what is this condition called?

It's called the dysfunction of the belch syndrome, and it can be extremely painful. A recent article in *Gastroneurology* recounts the case of a 25-year-old woman who complained of an incapacitating chest pain. She went from doctor to doctor, unable to get any substantial diagnosis. None of them could find any organic cause of her chest pain. She was told she had a psychocardiac neurosis and was probably recommended for psychotherapy, but she finally got a doctor to diagnose her condition correctly. Her upper esophageal sphincter was malfunctioning so that gas could not escape; the gas would remain trapped within the esophagus for so long that the esophagus, it appeared, would mistake it for a stuck piece of food and clamp down on it, trying to push it down into the stomach. The upward pressure of the gas against the downward pressure of the esophagus push was like a hot air balloon in a trash compactor; the pain was quite possibly more debilitating than that of a massive coronary.

Why do you think it was so difficult for all those doctors to diagnose that condition?

Most likely because it just never occurred to these doctors. They were probably so concerned about making sure she was not having a heart attack that they did not stop to consider this or any other esophagus-related condition. They may not have been listening carefully enough to the patient, or perhaps the patient was unable fully to communicate to the doctors, given the intensity of her chest pain. Knowing what you now know, of course, you might possibly avoid going to ten different doctors with this condition. If your doctor cannot find anything physically wrong with you, ask yourself, "Have I belched lately? Have I belched measurably less than usual?" If the answers are "no" and "yes," ask your doctor to fluoroscope and X-ray your esophagus. Of course, there is no guarantee you will resolve the mystery but if the pain is really bad, it is probably worth a try.

What can be done about it?

Your doctor may need to prescribe motor coordination medicines such as Reglan in order to relax this upper esophageal sphincter muscle. You may also require pain killers temporarily, but most important are preventive measures to decrease the chances of recurrence. If you discover that you do have a predisposition toward this syndrome, it is probably a good idea to lighten up on the production of gas in your stomach. Stress, overeating, eating too quickly, and gum chewing are common causes of excess gas. Soda pop and other carbonated beverages are the most obvious gaseous items in the average American diet, since most get their carbonation from injected CO_2 gas. Foods that tend to produce excess gas in most people include too many fruits and vegetables (especially onions, garlic, and *cruciferous vegetables* in the cabbage family such as broccoli, cabbage, and cauliflower); beans; legumes; milk and other dairy products; and wheat products—though virtually anything can probably be said to cause gas in someone somewhere.

Other than the pain, how serious is this condition?

There aren't really enough reports of prolonged cases to give an accurate answer, but my guess is that, other than the pain (which should not be understated and is very important because it can mask a coronary), this syndrome is probably not life-threatening or very serious. Not nearly as serious as, say, an esophageal rupture.

An esophageal rupture? Dare I ask what that is?
It is the tearing of the wall of the esophagus. If not treated, it can cause an infection. If the infection is not treated, hemorrhaging and possibly a life-threatening infection can occur. Sometimes the tear causes unrelenting hiccups, sometimes there is the vomiting of blood (this is referred to as the Mallory-Weiss syndrome and occurs more often in those who abuse alcohol). Esophageal rupture, whatever the symptoms, is probably a medical emergency.

What's the cause?
Most of the time these ruptures—which are relatively rare—are spontaneous and happen for unknown reasons. The explainable ruptures are usually the result of a swallowed piece of solid matter that tears or pokes a hole in the esophagus lining. Under these circumstances X rays will usually find chicken bones, fish bones, or other splintered meat bones. I would suspect, however, that, if you were to interview every internist and emergency room radiologist, you could compile a significant list of objects (it may not include a kitchen sink but may very well include certain parts of one) that have, at one time, ended up inside someone's esophagus. Probably the most bizarre object I ever discovered under these circumstances was inside a boy who couldn't have been more than ten years old. He was in such pain his mother had to hold him still as I listened to his heart and his breathing, which sounded normal. It took several assistants to hold him down on the X-ray table. The X rays showed an axle with two wheels from a toy railroad car. I have heard from several colleagues of mine about patients who, having had a little too much to drink, consumed martini olives with the toothpick still in them or even the sharpened end of a pencil and then

woke up in the middle of the night with no memory of this blunder but with a chest pain that felt like a heart attack. In this case the mistaken self-diagnosis proves beneficial given the seriousness of a ruptured or pierced esophagus.

How do you fix the rupture?

If it is caused by a foreign object, that object must first be identified, located, and removed. The rupture itself is repaired surgically.

How common are these sometimes spontaneous and potentially fatal ruptures?

Fortunately, they are quite rare. A more common—and less serious—complication of the esophagus is ulceration.

What is an ulcerated esophagus?

It is a hole or an erosion in the lining of the esophagus, not from tearing but from burning. Long-term, untreated heartburn can result in these esophageal ulcers. So can swallowing too many pills without water or some fluid. Pills, if taken without accompanying liquid, can get stuck in the esophagus, dissolve slowly, and burn. Bulimics—those people who induce vomiting as a form of weight control—are purging not only food but HCl, which can, over a long period, ravage the walls of the esophagus, potentially causing ulcerations. (It also, incidentally, causes rotting of the teeth.)

How are these ulcers treated?

Surgery is rarely needed. Usually, esophageal ulcers will heal on their own with medication. You must then deal with their cause to prevent recurrence. Tissue damage to the esophagus can be a real health hazard. It may even be a cause of esophageal motility disorders.

Esophageal motility disorders?

This is an abnormality in *peristalsis* (the direction of the motion of the esophagus), which is supposed to be downward during eating and upward during the letting out of gas. The direction of this motion is what allows us to eat lying down or in a spaceship without the benefit of gravity to move the food to the stomach. The disorder occurs when the esophagus muscle begins contracting in both directions at the same time. These counter-contractions collide with each other, causing a chest pain that can be debilitating. This pain usually occurs while swallowing, though it can happen at any time. Sometimes there can be total effective obstruction so that nothing can pass through the esophagus. Any piece of food still present is now stuck—unleashing acute pain and other complications.

What kind of other complications?

Food may be regurgitated into the lungs during sleep or any semiconscious state, causing infection and pneumonia.

How do you get the piece of food out before this happens?

The easiest way is for your doctor to dilate the sphincter, creating an artificially large opening. This can sometimes allow stuck pieces of food to pass into the stomach.

How does my doctor dilate my sphincter?

Nitroglycerin under the tongue can be helpful, as can calcium channel blocker medicines, which manipulate calcium ion exchanges and cause dilation to occur (they do not block the absorption of dietary calcium). Unfortunately, these medicines can also cause heartburn because they relax the sphincter muscles of the esophagus. Your doctor will have to weigh that against the urgency of the trapped food of a motility disorder.

What if dilation doesn't work?

Then the food must be surgically removed, most likely with an endoscope.

Is there any treatment for esophageal motility disorder? Any way to prevent recurrence?

There is no surefire treatment yet established, though esophagus motion may be encouraged by Bethanechol, a drug therapy you must follow under the supervision of a doctor.

What, other than esophageal ulcers, causes the esophageal motility disorder?

We're not even sure of the ulcer connection, but there is a generally held suspicion that any tissue damage to the esophagus muscle may be a cause of this illness. It is also believed that esophageal motility disorder can be symptomatic of multiple sclerosis and other neurological diseases. There is also a disease known as nutcracker esophagus syndrome, in which an area of the esophagus muscle becomes nonfunctional even though there is no tissue damage. Its cause is not yet known.

Any other esophagus-related causes of chest pain?

Diffuse esophageal noneffective spasms (which is a fancy way of saying that the esophagus is not doing what it is supposed to) can occur for no apparent reason, causing substernal pain that can often wake the patient in the middle of the night. Drinking cold water worsens the pain; a patient will often do this, believing his or her pain is that of heartburn. These spasms can lead to esophageal motility disorders.

There is also an illness called *achalasia*, which is characterized by a reduction or cessation of the peristalsis function. The sphincter muscle that allows food and fluid into the stomach fails to relax. This failure causes painful swallowing and often a feeling of fullness in the chest—usually the midchest area, as the result of food that gets "hung up"— which can become painful.

What kind of pain?

Often it is substernal chest pain, but the pain can radiate to the neck, arms, and back and is usually—though not necessarily—the result of swallowing. Cold beverages precipitate this pain most often, since they cause the muscle to contract. There may also be spasms of the esophagus brought on by antiperistalsis—the muscle contractions moving in the wrong direction. Sometimes this condition can bring on the sensation of having a lump form in the throat, and this lump is often misdiagnosed as heart angina.

What causes this problem?

Achalasia is caused by a loss of proper nerve tissue functioning in the area for unknown reasons.

How is it treated?

Sometimes a pneumatic dilator is used to dilate the esophagus, splitting the muscle fibers in the clenched sphincter and making it more flexible, which allows food and liquid to pass through. Some of the calcium channel blocker drugs, such as nifedipine, seem to lower pressure in the sphincter contraction. Sometimes surgery is needed to repair the nonfunctional tissue. Diagnosis can be made using X ray, fluoroscopy, and an endoscope.

Does that take care of esophageal-related chest pain?

Not quite. Chest pain can occur as the result of an infection of the esophagus—for reasons previously mentioned and for other reasons. Chest pain may also be symptomatic of esophageal viruses such as herpes. Tumors, benign or malignant, can grow on the esophagus, resulting from Barrett's esophagus and achalasia as well as other known and unknown reasons. These tumors, if cancerous, can be removed or contained if caught early (another reason why responding to a chest pain can save your life).

In addition, there are, as always in medicine, the unknown or yet-to-be-known esophageal syndromes. In fact, there is a label for all not-yet-understood conditions of this sort. They are simply called irritable esophagus syndrome. If your doctor tells you that's what you have, it probably means that medical science has yet to discover what it is that you have. Most of these conditions usually are treatable with medication.

What about the treatment of recurrent infections?

Antibiotic therapy will sometimes work eventually. Sometimes, however, the patient is immune-suppressed.

You mean AIDS?

Not necessarily. For every person suffering from Acquired Immune Deficiency Syndrome, there are probably many more people whose immunity is suppressed because they are overweight, malnourished, overly stressed, unloved, and out of shape. Many of the suggestions I make in the *Answering Pain with Action* section of this book can help increase your immunity against infections, viruses, and even some cancers.

With all these different esophageal conditions, how would I know what I have?

You wouldn't. Only a doctor would. That's why I question the responsibility of any television commercial that shows a guy clutching his breastbone while his wife serves up the antacid. How does she know he's not having counter-contractions, trapped gas, or a tie-clip—or a tumor—in his esophagus? Furthermore, when an ulcer or lesion or any inflammation, viral or otherwise, heals in the esophagus it can leave a stricture. This means that a part of the esophagus muscle is stuck in a contracted position. Swallowing can become difficult and painful, and food won't pass properly into the stomach. Esophagus strictures require mechanical stretching with a dilator and sometimes require reconstructive surgery of the esophagus muscle. For that reason alone, the treatment for esophagus-related chest pain is *not* on a drugstore shelf.

Stomach-Related Chest Pain

How could a problem in the stomach feel like a heart attack?

Although the pain of any stomach illness is *usually* felt in the abdominal area, under certain circumstances in certain people, many stomach ailments have been known to cause a pain that is felt in the chest. This is probably a consequence of the relative proximity of the two sets of nerve pathways that deliver pain messages from the stomach to the brain and from the heart to the brain. Like the telephone company's microcircuitry, sometimes it inadvertently misreads a signal and connects you with the wrong number. Some stomach upsets can cause rapid heartbeats, which in turn can cause chest pain.

Which stomach condition is most likely to cause a chest pain?

Based on my medical practice, I would have to say *gastritis,* an inflammation—itis—of the stomach—gastr(ic).

What causes the inflammation?

It turns out to be our old friend hydrochloric acid.

29

What about that protective mucous lining in the stomach?

It's a natural wonder, but it's not impervious. In some people there are a number of factors that wear away a specific area of this protective shield, allowing HCl—as well as another digestive enzyme called pepsin—to burn the stomach wall.

Alcohol, in excess, is infamous for this. In some folks even just a little firewater can ignite a case of gastritis, potentially causing a chest pain.

Another common irritant for some are those consumables deriving from weeds, such as tobacco and marijuana. Whether smoked, chewed, or sucked on, they are capable of sparking gastritis and chest pain. It seems that certain chemicals in weeds, when dissolved by saliva, can irritate the stomach lining.

Drinking too much soda pop can also irritate the stomach lining because sodas contain phosphoric acid and carbonation. So can overdoing spices. Some over-the-counter and prescription drugs are often associated with gastritis. According to a recent medical theory, aspirin and other common painkillers—such as those of the nonsteroidal antiinflammatory ibuprofen group (such as Motrin, Advil, and many others)—shut off the manufacture of prostaglandins (hormones essential to the maintenance of the stomach's integrity). Many other drugs—in fact, *any* drug—can upset someone's stomach, causing an abdominal or chest pain.

Stress—resulting from emotional pressures or illnesses such as viral and other severe infections, lung disease, and cancer—can also compromise an intact stomach lining. So can bacteria, such as strep and staphylococci.

There are two versions of gastritis: acute and chronic.

Are the causes known to be different for the two versions?

Yes, though there is some overlap.

Short-term, acute gastritis usually occurs from a sudden severe stress, such as the burning of indigestion, a trauma such as the ingestion of lye or other abrasive, surgery, coma, kidney failure, head injury, or adrenal gland problem. In fact, there is an illness called epidemic gastritis, in which the stomach is, for unknown reasons, infected with a bacteria called Campylobacter pyloris.

Chronic gastritis can result from habitual overuse of aspirin and other drugs, infections, viruses, overindulgence in high-acid foods and alcohol, gland atrophy, and a variety of unknown reasons that tend to occur more in people over the age of 45. One such gastritis of unknown origins is called Ménétrièr's disease and is characterized by a shrinking of the stomach lining, which initiates pain in the *epigastrium* (the upper stomach, beneath the sternum) and lower sternal (breastbone) areas.

Is either of the versions more likely to cause a chest pain?

No. Both are usually felt in the abdominal area, but either can cause chest pain.

Are there any significant characteristics of the chest pain?

It is usually at the lower mid-line center of the torso—between the chest and abdomen—but sometimes can radiate to the left nipple area. Often, but not always, it is associated with nausea. Sometimes drinking cold water can instigate the chest pain or make it worse. There can be vomiting as well as back pain. Also, it can begin with a pain in the epigastrium and then move to the chest area.

How is it treated?

Short-term acute gastritis is usually treated in the hospital with antacid medications, a diet low in acid-producing foods, and fluids. If there is hemorrhaging, it may seem appropriate to close an artery surgically with an endoscope (an investigative instrument with lamp and lenses thin enough to pass through the mouth and down into the esophagus) and cautery. Surgical removal of part of the stomach may also be considered if the internal bleeding does not cease. Researchers are now experimenting with the group of prostaglandin *E* types to determine whether injected doses are as effective as those normally produced within the body. *Prostaglandins* are hormones, some of which protect the integrity of the stomach. So far, the research looks good; there is even evidence that these prostaglandins may be effective in lowering the production rate of stomach acids.

A common folk remedy you may have heard of and one I do *not* recommend is sodium bicarbonate (a.k.a. baking soda). Although it may work to settle the stomach and soothe chest or abdominal pain, sodium bicarbonate can also increase blood pressure and chronic use can increase the risk of kidney degeneration and heart disease.

Treatment for chronic gastritis is dictated by its cause if known. Often it's treated much the same way as acute gastritis, with medicine and alteration of diet.

Of course, the only really sound way to approach the problem is to get your doctor to prescribe some preventive measures. Decreasing alcohol consumption, eliminating tobacco products and other aggravators from your diet, and trading in the perverse benefits of stress for some no-nonsense quality health are starters. The long-term effects of chronic gastritis (or even too many bouts of short-term gastritis) are pain, suffering, anemia, and possibly stomach cancer. And, like all other causes of noncardiac chest pain, it can render you too tolerant of chest pain.

What other stomach illnesses can cause chest pain?

Stomach ulcers, like gastritis, are generally associated with abdominal pain but can cause burning in the chest.

Did you say ulcers—as in more than one kind?

Both peptic and duodenal ulcers can result in chest pain. They share many characteristics, but they differ in location: peptic means within the stomach, duodenal refers to the pylorus valve and its immediate vicinity between the stomach and the first part of the intestine, known as the *duodenum*.

There is not yet absolute certainty about the cause of either kind of ulcer. In some cases, there may be no cause; it might be something that just happens to some people. Ulcers do, in many instances, appear to result from an excess of stomach acid and the digestive enzyme pepsin. These excesses may be associated with bacterial infections, such as Campylobacter pyloris, and imbalances of mucus, prostaglandin, pepsin, and HCl. You may be genetically predisposed to ulcers. You may also be at risk for ulcers if you are a chronic user of aspirin.

Researchers have devoted much speculation to the connection between emotional and environmental stress and ulcers. Ulcer victims are often people with an angry disposition, full of frustration, often seemingly in conflict or riddled with unresolved guilts. As the theory goes, these unsettling emotions (or any other emotional imbalances) can increase acid production in the stomach.

Many studies have also linked smoking, alcohol, tea, coffee (and other substances containing caffeine), sodas, and anything else containing phosphoric acid, as well as a variety of medicines (including aspirin, cortisone, analgesics, and antiinflammatory drugs) to peptic and duodenal ulcers. These ulcers may also be a response to a failure of the body to produce prostaglandins or protective mucus. They may also result from herpes, other viruses, and some bacteria. There may even be an autoimmune form of ulcer. *Autoimmune disorders* are illnesses caused by an immune system gone haywire.

What kind of chest pain can result?

Usually the chest pain of ulcer is characterized by burning or gnawing in the chest mid-line area (substernal, between the shoulder blades in the back). Of course, it is likely to be accompanied by a similar pain in the stomach area. Pain most often occurs at night, early in the morning, or any time the stomach has been empty for a number of hours. As long as there is food in the stomach, excess acid should not attack the stomach wall. It is probably for this reason that many people describe their ulcer pain as a hunger pang. For some people the pain of an ulcer is noticeably worse during the spring and fall, though no one has been able to put a conclusive finger on why. Any high-acid foods (watch out for those pickles!) will increase the pain of an ulcer; for this reason, the *cause* of ulcers is mistakenly attributed to these spicy, tart, or sour foods.

What do I do about the pain?

You don't do anything about it because there is no way you could possibly know that what you're feeling is an ulcer. In fact, a physical exam may very well not show any such evidence. Even an upper gastrointestinal tract X ray may not be accurate. The most reliable diagnostic tool for discovering ulcers is an endoscope.

If a duodenal or peptic ulcer is found, most doctors will prescribe one of the many commonly used medications, such as Tagamet, Zantac, Carafate, or Pepcid, or an antacid (for treatment of ulcers their medicinal benefits probably outweigh the potential side effects, at least in the short run). A recent study found that combined dosages of Carafate and either Zantac or Tagamet helps mucous cells to recoat the stomach, repairing ulcer damage in some people. If your doctor does prescribe Carafate for you, make sure *not* to take it with food since food seems to hinder its effectiveness. Prostaglandin therapies, still experimental and under review by researchers, may help in the treatment of ulcers in much the same way if the Food and Drug Administration (FDA) ever approves them.

I heard somewhere that licorice is a good ulcer remedy.

My grandmother used it all the time. It's a famous folk remedy. Allegedly, a chemical contained in licorice called glycyrrhizic acid (or one of its breakdown products) helps heal ulcers. Its efficacy has not been scientifically proven, and there is speculation that licorice (eaten as candy or in the pure root form) may elevate blood pressure—not a good trade-off.

What about "plop plop fizz fizz"?

Calcium carbonate, the favorite over-the-counter remedy, for which Madison Avenue is paid generously each year in advertising its various brand names, is not such a good remedy for ulcers. It may give temporary relief, but in about 45 minutes (sometimes an hour or two) an acid rebound can cause the return of pain, sometimes at an even more intense level. The same is, unfortunately, true for many people who try to treat ulcers with milk. The temporary relief is not worth the long-term pain and potential worsening of the condition. Until recently, milk was used as a bedtime snack to prevent middle-of-the-night ulcer pain. Now, most doctors would probably recommend a banana, which seems to settle the stomach without causing an acid rebound.

Any other foods I should emphasize or avoid?

Yes, there are some dietary considerations, though diet is no longer regarded as the cornerstone of ulcer treatment. Your doctor will probably recommend a low-carbohydrate, moderate-fat, high-protein regimen. Since you probably bought this book because you don't want to die of heart disease, get the bulk of your protein from fresh fish or beans and legumes, revise your fat intake from moderate to low, and avoid saturated fats. There is evidence that saturated fat (which I will discuss later in greater detail) is an irritant to most ulcers.

In my practice I also suggest a high-fiber diet; some new research points to fiber's possible role in healing an ulcerated stomach. Significant amounts of *betacarotene* (the dietary substance from which our bodies derive vitamin A), which is found in all yellow vegetables and a variety of other foods, can help support the integrity of the mucous cell lining and the growth of these mucous cells necessary to protect the stomach lining. Vitamin C, taken after each meal, also seems to build better intracellular "cement" and, in general, to encourage the healing process. Ulcer patients should take their vitamin C in the buffered (not the acid) form, which they will be more able to tolerate, and should *never* take vitamin C on an empty stomach.

I also urge my ulcer patients to eliminate or reduce drastically alcohol, vinegar, high-acid fruits, sodas, refined sugars and refined carbohydrates, and cigarette smoking in their diets. Eating less more often—up to six small meals per day—can also keep the stomach occupied more often while being taxed less.

In the long run, you need to control anxiety, stress, and other high-impact, low-benefit emotions not only because of their probable link to ulcers but also because they are a major contributing cause of heart disease and heart attack.

What if I'm stoic and don't do anything?

That's not stoic, it's masochistic! If left untreated, an ulcer can perforate—actually breaking open a small piece of the intestine or the stomach wall—or begin to hemorrhage. In either case, it's a medical emergency.

The pain of a perforated ulcer is usually upper abdominal, but it can also manifest itself as a chest pain—sudden, severe, and unrelenting, often growing worse with each movement. It can be accompanied by a very fast heart rate and a drop in blood pressure. If that doesn't get you on the phone to the paramedics, you're not stoic *or* masochistic, you're crazy!

The symptoms of a bleeding ulcer include vomiting blood, fainting, sweating, diarrhea, and black, tarry stool. Immediate hospitalization is a must. In fact, any ulcer that is not relieved either by eating or by medication is a reason to get immediate medical attention.

Okay, okay, doctor, you've scared me out of my stoicism. What's the treatment for ulcers?

Most peptic and duodenal ulcers do not require surgery. They are treated with medication along with recommendations for diet and lifestyle changes. About 75% should heal within five to six weeks. Initial treatment, in my opinion, should last from six to eight weeks. During this time, your doctor will keep a close watch on your blood count. Iron, B_{12}, and folic acid deficiency anemias can develop in ulcer patients because of poor vitamin and mineral absorption, as well as from the side effects of some ulcer medications.

If treatment fails, your doctor will probably change drugs and/or dosage, combine medications, and—this is almost a must—investigate potential other, underlying medical conditions. At least 2% of all stomach ulcers may be symptomatic of stomach cancer; ulcers can also be an early warning of pancreatic cancer. As a last resort, your doctor may consider surgery.

What kind of surgery?

It usually involves cutting the nerves that are producing the excess stomach acid and, if necessary, closing the sites of bleeding. As with any surgery, always get a second opinion before laying yourself on the table.

How would I know if I'm among the 2% with stomach cancer?

Endoscopy is a valuable diagnostic procedure because it can enable your physician to find cancer of the stomach when present. Since, like all tools of medicine (including the eyes and other senses of the doctor), the endoscope is imperfect, it is always a good idea to have your doctor take another look if, after eight weeks, a stomach ulcer does not respond to regular treatment. There are also stool tests that can reveal the presence of cancer in the stomach. If, after 12 weeks and several endoscopies (and stool tests), no cancer is found but the pain persists as does the ulcer, you may wish to consider explorative surgery and biopsy to make sure there is no inconspicuous cancer.

Early symptoms of stomach cancer include a *diffuse pain* (pain in no specific location) in the chest or abdominal area after eating, painful swallowing, a feeling of fullness after you have just barely started eating, bloating, nausea, and vomiting. Anemia and low blood sugar are common symptoms of stomach cancer. The more severe symptoms include increased heart rate (because of anemia) leading to an *ischemic heart* (a heart lacking enough oxygen for its own cell processes per unit of time and contraction) and causing angina (heart pain). Stomach cancer, if not dealt with, can even produce a heart attack.

Is stomach cancer treatable?

If detected early enough, yes. It can be surgically removed.

Any other stomach conditions that cause chest pain?

There is an illness called Zollinger-Ellison syndrome. It is characterized by an excess of *gastrin* (a gastric enzyme in the blood). It usually leads to recurring peptic ulcers or to ulcers in more unusual places (in the middle of the intestines, for example), though a diffuse and often vague pain can be felt in the chest area. It is usually accompanied by diarrhea. This condition is most common among men ages 35 to 65 and is often associated with parathyroid gland disease, in which a tumor of the intestines or pancreas causes excess secretion of parathyroid hormone, which controls calcium metabolism and can cause the blood calcium level to rise abnormally.

How is it treated?

With surgery or very high doses of ulcer medicines. As with most ulcers and other stomach illnesses, early treatment, which begins with your response to your chest pain, is critical.

Pancreas-Related Chest Pain

What is a pancreas and what does it do for me?

The pancreas is a gland located directly behind the stomach. It digests fat (which it does by secreting lipase enzyme) and aids in the digestion of protein and amino acids (which it does by secreting trypsin enzyme).

And how might mine cause me a chest pain?

There are two illnesses that might do this. The first one is pancreatitis, which is an inflammation of the pancreas. The resulting pain is usually mid-abdominal but can also strike in the upper posterior chest, between the shoulder blades. Or it can be a dull pain in the epigastrium or it can hit you in the back. In about 70% of cases it is accompanied by nausea and vomiting. At first its pain may resemble that of a peptic ulcer.

What's the cause?

In simple terms, it is a leak in the pancreatic cells around its own structure. The pancreatic digestive enzymes—the ones meant to break down fats and help break down proteins in the large intestines—never get that far. They leak into the tissue of the pancreas itself and thus the pancreas begins to digest itself.

What makes this happen?

It can be a reaction to drugs such as thiazide *diuretics* (used to reduce body fluid and lower blood pressure) and *cortisone* (a painkiller commonly used against arthritis), alcohol, viruses, parasites, gallbladder disease, and penetrating ulcers. Fat and alcohol have been known to make the inflammation—and the pain—worse.

What's the treatment?

Immediate hospitalization and intensive care under the supervision of a doctor. It is a medical emergency of the first order that, if not dealt with, can lead to fatal hemorrhaging, low blood pressure, *pericardial effusion* (bleeding between the lining of the heart and the heart itself), and other heart complications.

What's the other pancreatic disorder that causes chest pain?

Well, if you can believe it, pancreatitis is the one you'd rather have. The other illness is cancer of the pancreas, which can cause upper chest pain, diffuse pain, and back pain (which will often be at least temporarily relieved by sitting up and leaning forward). Depression is a common symptom, which, as we will later discuss, can cause a chest pain of the most intense magnitude. Depression, in fact, can be the only early symptom of a pancreatic cancer, though there may also be a mild anemia.

Any known causes?

It is the fourth most common kind of cancer. Cigarette smoking is believed to be at or near the top of the list of causes, as well as diets high in fat. There are some in the medical profession who believe there is a link between coffee consumption and the risk of pancreatic cancer, although this is still controversial. There also may be a connection between working in oil refineries or around gasoline for a long period of time and this kind of cancer.

What's the treatment?

There isn't much that can be done about this particular form of cancer, which is another good reason to quit smoking, reduce fat and coffee consumption, and take extra precautions against the potential toxic effects of petroleum products if you are significantly exposed to them in your work environment.

I must add, however, that the likelihood of any chest pain being the result of pancreatic cancer is sufficiently small enough that this information should not initiate dread or apathy, given that most other causes of chest pain are treatable if dealt with in a timely manner.

Gallbladder-Related Chest Pain

What's a gallbladder and what is it supposed to do?

The gallbladder stores *bile,* a digestive enzyme produced in the liver. When this bile is needed to help digest fats, the gallbladder contracts, issuing the bile into the duodenum (the first part of the small intestine). It works on demand. Every time you eat some fat, you put the gallbladder to work.

How does it cause a chest pain?

The most commonly known reason is *gallstones,* which are solidified deposits of bile and cholesterol. *Cholelithiasis* (the medical name for gallstones) usually causes pain in the upper right abdomen under the bottom rib. Because of course this is only inches from the center of the chest, the pain can be interpreted as a chest pain. Sometimes the pain is felt in the tip of the right shoulder blade or the mid-upper back. Sometimes the pain is only felt at night or near early morning.

What causes gallstones?

No one is absolutely sure. Excess fats and cholesterol would seem to increase anyone's risk, though some people seem more vulnerable than others. These stones are most common in women; between 10% and 20% of all women between the ages of 50 and 60 have these gallstones. Pregnancy increases a woman's chances of having them. Obesity and *diabetes mellitus* (sugar-related diabetes) increase anyone's risk of gallstones.

And the treatment?

Sometimes the stones, if small enough, can be dissolved with certain new chemicals inserted by tube into the gallbladder. For gallstones between about 20 and 50 millimeters in size, chenodeoxycholic acid and ursodeoxycholic acid, taken orally, seem to eliminate them successfully. The stones are usually gone within three months, but one continues the medicine for an additional three months to help prevent recurrence.

Another new procedure, useful for single stones of 30 millimeters or less, is *lithotripsy* (a treatment that passes sound waves through the body to break up gallstones). Between these two new approaches, researchers are finding that most individual stones of sufficiently small size can be treated without gallbladder surgery.

What are the risks of nontreatment?

Complications of gallbladder disease include infections. These happen if the gallbladder becomes unable, because of a large stone, to empty its contents—which can then turn stale—and the blood supply in the gallbladder, which helps protect it from infection, is greatly reduced. If not dealt with, gallstones can also cause *empyema* (a collection of pus that cannot drain and that can result in gangrene) of the gallbladder, a medical emergency requiring major surgery. People with gallstones seem to be more vulnerable to coronary heart disease, yet another reason for early treatment and preventive measures.

Are there any other ways in which the gallbladder can cause chest pain?

As with almost anything, there are potentially unknown links between the gallbladder and chest pain. For example, cancer of the gallbladder, a very uncommon form of cancer, is difficult to diagnose because less than half of all cases have any kind of pain and, of that portion, there are no solid estimates of how many experience chest pain. Almost all cases are associated with *jaundice* (yellowing of the skin and the whites of the eyes, lassitude, and loss of appetite), weight loss, fever, chills, and diarrhea or constipation. Treatment, as with most cancers, involves surgical removal of the cancer, if possible, and radiation or chemotherapy, if not.

Pulmonary-Related Chest Pain

Do I detect a movement upward in the anatomy?

You're quite right. The two lungs flank the heart. They are the central organ of the respiratory system and their most important function is to draw in air so that the blood circulating through the arteries, membranes, and capillaries of the lungs can absorb oxygen. They feed oxygen into the heart through the atrium to the ventricle, where it is pumped through the arteries of the entire body. Cells then absorb the oxygen and return carbon dioxide to the blood, which then returns, through the veins, to the lungs to be exhaled back into the earth's oxygen cycle. It is estimated that each day the average human breathes in 30 pounds—which is about 3,500 gallons—of oxygen. It is also estimated that we cannot live without oxygen for more than about five minutes. The breathing process, like our circulatory system, is automatic.

What lung disorders cause chest pain?

Because of their proximity to the heart, virtually any disorder of the lungs can result in a chest pain. Because of the heart's constant need for fresh oxygen, all respiratory illnesses, pulmonary or otherwise, should be taken seriously and considered a potential medical emergency, be it pneumonia or a *pulmonary embolus*.

What's a pulmonary embolus?

It's a clot—usually a blood clot, though it can, in fact, be fat from bone trauma or any lodged piece of organic material—in a lung artery or capillary. Usually they occur singly, and for most people they are an isolated problem. About 600,000 people experience pulmonary emboli every year.

Where do they come from?

Virtually anywhere in the body. Often the clot will come all the way from veins in the leg, deep veins in the pelvis, varicose veins anywhere in the body; it will circulate all the way to a pulmonary artery or capillary that is too narrow for the clot to pass through. Blood pooling is a common cause.

What's blood pooling?

It's the collecting of blood in a specific location, from which it cannot move on because of blocked circulatory plumbing, usually from plugged or compressed arteries. Blood pooling can occur anywhere in the lung or in the rest of the body.

Are there other causes of pulmonary embolus?

Yes, quite a few. Pulmonary embolus can result from obesity, pregnancy, varicosities, and a variety of blood clotting disorders such as *polycythemia* (excessive platelets and red blood cells). Blood clots can form as the reaction to major (and some minor) surgery. Blood clots can also be an early symptom of lung, breast, or intestinal cancer and can help lead to a doctor's early diagnosis of these life-threatening but treatable malignancies. There are also some rare hereditary blood clotting illnesses, which cause a failure of the body's *antithrombotic* (anti-platelet clotting) proteins or a deficiency of clotting and anticlotting body chemicals.

But you say pulmonary emboli are not necessarily blood clots?

That's right. In some cases, they can be air bubbles in the blood.

Air bubbles? How does that happen?

Any gaping wound exposing a piece of bone to surface air or an injected syringe can allow the formation of air bubbles. Emboli can also be caused by fat cells and, in rare cases, stray cancer cells or clumps. Some intravenous drug users have even been known to suffer a pulmonary embolus from talc or cornstarch that was presumably mixed with the heroin or cocaine.

What kind of chest pain are we talking about?

About 88% of all pulmonary emboli cause chest pain; about 85% of that pain is *pleuritic pain* (sudden sharp or grating chest pain usually worsened with each breath and accompanied by shortness of breath). It can also be accompanied by fear, perspiring, coughing (sometimes with blood), fever, swelling of body parts, and, in about 10% of all cases, faintness. About half of all pulmonary emboli cause increased pulse. About 90% cause rapid heartbeat, which is often the cause of a chest pain. Light-headedness may also occur.

You say 85% is pleuritic pain. What about the other 15%?

The rest *can* be any kind of chest pain, though it is usually confined to the substernal area. For this reason a pulmonary embolus can be mistaken for asthma, a fractured rib, or *postherpetic neuritis* (a complication of shingles).

How is a pulmonary embolus treated?

First your doctor has to make a diagnosis, which can be tricky because the illness is similar to *pleurisy* (a disease of the lining of the lungs), pneumonia, cancer, or heart attack. Diagnosis is usually made with X rays and various scans, as well as EKGs, *pulmonary arteriography* (a dye study of the pulmonary blood vessels), and arterial blood gas measurements (since pulmonary emboli often cause a drop in the percentage of oxygen dissolved in the blood).

Once diagnosis is made, your doctor may try one of several methods of anticoagulation to get rid of the obstructing clot. Often the simplest method is to dissolve the clots with heparin injections. Dipyridamole or Coumadin may also be used to stop future clotting. If these procedures are not in order or fail, analgesics often relieve pain while oxygen is administered (to relieve the demands of the compromised lung) until the embolus can be dealt with. Thrombolysis may be the next treatment of choice, using intravenous clot-dissolving chemicals; however, I advise pregnant women and people just recovered from surgery against such treatment. If nothing else works, the pulmonary embolus must be surgically removed.

Pulmonary emboli are a serious problem. It is estimated that, of the 600,000 people who get them every year, 200,000—one in three—die as a result. Pulmonary emboli can lead to many serious complications, including heart disease and, in from 10% to 15% of cases, death.

Anything I can do to prevent pulmonary emboli in the first place?

Sure. If you're overweight, lose weight. If you wear stockings (and whether you do, Mr. Strauss, is none of my business), wear elastic, not nylon, stockings. If there is a recurring problem with blood clots, you may want to talk to your doctor about anticoagulation medicines, like heparin and Coumadin. When blood clots become recurrent, they pose a serious health problem, and your doctor may consider ligating (closing) your *inferior vena cava.*

What's an inferior vena cava?

It's the major vein returning blood to the cardiac pulmonary system.

If you close it, how does blood flow back to the heart and lungs?

The circulatory system detours it through alternate venous routes. This is radical surgery, and you should consider it only if recurring blood clots put you at risk for stroke or if they persistently cause pulmonary hypertension.

What is pulmonary hypertension?

High blood pressure within the lungs. High blood pressure means that there is more blood flowing through the limited capacity of veins, arteries, and capillaries. Hypertension occurs when too much blood tries to flow through the entire body's circulatory system, putting a strain on the heart muscle. With pulmonary hypertension, the strain is placed on the lungs, though the pain can feel identical to the pain of heart disease.

What, other than pulmonary embolus, causes pulmonary hypertension?

An overload of blood to the right side of the heart can cause high blood pressure in the pulmonary artery. So can chronic vascular (blood vessel) inflammation and closure or spasms of pulmonary blood vessels. Pulmonary hypertension can be symptomatic of *emphysema* (a disease of obstructed air flow) and heart disease, especially valve disorders, such as mitral stenosis, in which a valve allows blood to back up into the lung by failing to open and close properly.

Is the pain always like that of heart disease?

Never say always. The pain is usually similar to the pain of heart disease. Pulmonary hypertension is a syndrome of decreased oxygen, and any resulting pain is likely to mimic heart disease, but there are surely exceptions.

What is the treatment?

Treatment stems directly from diagnosis of the cause of the pulmonary hypertension. If the cause is a clot, get rid of the clot; if the problem is a heart valve, that valve may need to be replaced. Sometimes it is necessary to reduce total body fluid by decreasing dietary salt and using diuretics.

And if not treated?

Pulmonary hypertension puts a strain on the right ventricle, which pumps blood from the heart into the lungs, by making it pump with increasing force and higher pressure. Any pressure as high as 20 millimeters (which is a medical lab test and *not* a medical office procedure) is considered pulmonary hypertension. If that pressure rises to 40, the right side of the heart can begin to fail. When circulation fails, this can lead to complete heart failure, lung failure, and oxygen deprivation and can ultimately be fatal.

Anything I can do to prevent the condition?

Lots. Quit smoking and treat infections and respiratory and heart illnesses before pulmonary hypertension becomes a complication. If you are good to your lungs, you may also greatly reduce the risk of pulmonary abscess.

What's a pulmonary abscess?

It's an inflamed area composed of dead lung tissue, filled with pus, and surrounded by a fibrous capsule. It is localized, like any other kind of abscess—such as the kind a dentist might detect in your gum.

What's the cause?

Usually it is one of several things. Sometimes people will inhale some infected material through the upper airway and not cough it up. Often this happens to people who are either drunk or on tranquilizers or other sedative drug so that their cough reflex has been dulled. It can also happen during sleep, when all reflexes are dulled, or as the result of a stroke that completely eliminates reflexes.

What kind of infected material gets in the lung?

Usually it is something internal, for example, an infected postnasal drip. Rather than going down the esophagus, it will drip down the windpipe and into the lung. You don't always have to be drunk or sedated, because it can happen in your sleep. Sometimes, if you have reflux from the stomach, it can leap all the way through the esophagus, then back down the windpipe. The infected material can reach the lung and cause an abscess. Pulmonary abscesses are one of the hazards for those who work in jobs where they inhale dusts—such as coal, beryllium and other metals, and asbestos —all day. Some already present illnesses, such as Klebsiella pneumonia, can also cause an abscess. So can tuberculosis or fungus infections such as coccidioidomycosis, called Valley Fever because it is common in the California deserts.

What kind of chest pain does it inflict?

Usually it is a dull kind of pain that feels deep within the chest. Often the patient cannot pinpoint exactly where the pain is coming from, though the abscess itself is immobile. If, however, the abscess occurs on or near an area of *pleura* (lung lining), then the pain will most likely be sharp and related to breathing. Chills and fever often accompany this condition; it is an illness that usually sneaks up on you and can really wipe you out.

What's the treatment?

Treatment, as always, begins with a doctor's diagnosis. X rays can sometimes show an abscess. If not, a *bronchoscopy* (a look into the lung with a scope) will usually find the problem. A *CT scan* (a.k.a. cat scan, a computerized diagnostic imaging technique) can show the cavity of dead pustular tissue that is an abscess. Once the presence of an abscess has been established, your doctor may need to do cultures in order to know exactly what is growing in your lung before prescribing an appropriate treatment—penicillin or another antibiotic or antifungal. Cancer must be ruled out—or treated —as the underlying cause.

If I don't treat it?

Pulmonary abscesses can rupture and can spread the infection to more lung tissue. Such an abscess can also cause *sepsis* (general infections throughout the body with associated possible shock, once called "blood poisoning"), as well as arterial ruptures and potentially fatal arterial or venous hemorrhages. Part of the abscess can break off into an embolus, causing pulmonary hypertension and possibly leading to stroke. Lung abscesses can even lead to chronic lung disease. They are a serious medical condition. I hope you never get one, and if you do I hope you respect the potential danger.

What can I do to protect myself from getting a pulmonary abscess?

If you are in the habit of getting drunk or sedated, you might want to reconsider that particular habit. There are also ways in which we all can reduce our risk of infections in general. Always cover coughs and sneezes to avoid spreading bacteria and viruses—and insist that people close to you do the same. Use tissues, not hankies, and throw them away immediately after each use as if the soiled tissue were a ball of germs (which is exactly what it is). Then wash your hands. Talk to your doctor about immunization against the flu, talk to your pediatrician about immunizing your children, and you may even want to talk to your vet about putting your dog or cat on antibiotics.

So Fido doesn't get a pulmonary abscess?

No, so that you don't. You see, it is common for dogs and cats to carry streptococcal bacteria. The pet doesn't get infected by it but can give you the bacteria by licking you or licking their paws and touching you. A vet, whose job it is to treat the animal, isn't likely to prescribe medication for a bacteria that is not harming the dog or cat. It's up to you to tell the vet to check Fido or Mittens for streptococcus and, if necessary, prescribe antibiotics.

Other ways to help prevent respiratory infection are to breathe through your nose—which warms, humidifies, and filters air as the mouth does not—unless you are engaged in strenuous exercise. Keep the rooms in your house or office well-ventilated and relatively moist. To avoid dry mucous membranes and other sinus problems, use a humidifier if necessary and keep it clean. One possible indication that your home or work environment is too dry is if you frequently get an electric shock from touching objects. Also dust as often as possible. You would be revolted to see what microorganisms live on the edges of your books.

These preventive measures, by the way, will help decrease your risk of other illnesses, including pneumonia, which is possibly the most common cause of pulmonary chest pain.

Do people still get pneumonia?

Absolutely.

Haven't all those fancy new antibiotics wiped it out?

Not quite. Since the advent of so many new and varied antibiotics, if one does not work, others can be employed. Therefore, most bacterial infections are dealt with before they lead to pneumonia, but there is still cause for concern. Pneumonia is also caused by viruses, which don't respond to antibiotics. With millions of Americans suffering from suppressed immunity—not just from AIDS but from malnutrition, lack of exercise, and stress, pneumonia is making a comeback. In my own practice, in fact, I have noticed an increase in pneumonia as a cause of chest pain.

Pneumonia causes chest pain?

Usually it's a pleuritic pain on either the right or left side of the chest. The pain arises from the inflammation of the lining between the lung and the chest wall caused by the pneumonia. I have heard this pain described as feeling like sandpaper rubbed against the inside of the chest. Usually the pain is accompanied by fever and a cough, sometimes producing sputum that may be streaked with blood. Sometimes there is shortness of breath, sometimes drenching sweats and shivering chills. In most cases the symptoms add up to a sick patient, and thankfully it will usually inspire even the most stoic to seek medical attention. Interestingly, the very young and the very old, the most susceptible, are most likely to have what is called "walking pneumonia," in which they are dangerously sick but, for unknown reasons, don't feel it enough to get to a doctor (a terrific reason to have regular medical checkups).

How do you get pneumonia?
Most often it is still attributable to pneumococci bacteria. Sometimes streptococcal bacteria (that's the one you can get from your cat or dog), which is usually associated with strep throat, can wind up in the lungs and produce pneumonia. The pneumonia most often associated with AIDS is contracted through the Pneumocystis carinii parasite. Possibly the most serious kinds of pneumonia striking people *not* infected with the HIV virus are those caused by the staphylococcal bacteria, which is a very aggressive bacteria always present in the body though contained by a healthy immune system and which is usually the lingering effects of a really bad influenza. This pneumonia can be fatal. About one in three cases can lead to death, especially if not properly treated, and it is probably the most difficult to treat. It does not usually respond quickly to antibiotics, and so it is often difficult to find the right medicine with which to treat it. Some staphylococcal bacteria are totally resistant to penicillin and other of the more commonly used antibiotics. Pneumococcal pneumonia can be equally life-threatening but usually responds better to standard treatment. Streptococcal pneumonia is the least serious and most easily treated.

Some less common causes of pneumonia—and the related chest pain—include the bacteria Klebsiella and Pseudomonas. These bacteria tend to strike those who suffer from malnutrition, often the result of prolonged excessive use of alcohol, as well as people already suffering from Hodgkin's disease, *lymphoma* (malignancy of lymph tissue), the very old, and the very young. Legionnaire's disease can also cause pneumonia. So can another microorganism known as Mycoplasma, which, in contrast to most other kinds of lung infection, tends to progress at a much slower rate. The patient usually does not look or feel as sick. This can make its diagnosis more difficult, although there can sometimes be specific clues, such as neuropathy (electric feelings in the extremities) or a rash. It is generally a milder illness, but it can cause the same kind of chest pain. Any of the thousands of viruses in any population at a given time can potentially cause a pneumonia. Some specific viruses known to cause pneumonia are type A and type B influenza, Shanghai, Russian, Asian, rhino-, and adeno- viruses. Even measles and chicken pox can lead to viral pneumonia. It is now known that other herpes viruses, such as herpes simplex, can cause viral pneumonia, usually in those people suffering an immune disorder.

How are they all treated?

Antibiotics, most often penicillin or erythromycin, are taken along with bed rest. In the case of pneumonia caused by herpes virus or chicken pox, a drug called acyclovir may be used in treatment along with antibiotics. For staphylococcal pneumonia, special antibiotics like vancomycin often have to be taken intravenously in the hospital. Hospitalization may be necessary as the result of any kind of pneumonia, especially in those over 70, for whom the mortality rate from this illness is staggeringly high.

Diagnosis is, of course, crucial. This can be done using X rays, although they are not always necessary. Sometimes the symptoms, along with the lung sounds heard with a stethoscope, will tell your doctor all he or she needs to know.

It all sounds dreadful. What can I do to prevent all these lurking pneumonias?

There are a number of preventive measures you can take. Immunity plays a large part in virtually all the causes of pneumonia, which is why members of the same family can be exposed to the same viral or bacterial agents and yet not all will get sick. The immune system is a vast and ever-growing subject matter in medicine. It is already the subject of massive medical volumes. Briefly then, the immune system consists of the skin, the gastrointestinal tract, and protective blood cells known as macrophages, lymphocytes, and T cells. Countless medical studies have shown us that immunity—that is, our body's ability to defend itself against unfriendly invaders—is affected by nutrition, which should include the taking of vitamin and mineral supplements (see *The 50-Year Cholesterol and Hypertension Plan* for suggestions), exercise, and the elimination of some drugs and other substances. Immunity can be suppressed by stress, anxiety, and depression, and can probably be bolstered by loving relationships, laughter, and Mozart (or any music or art that is enjoyed). It can also be suppressed by cigarette smoking or excess alcohol consumption. A strong immunity is the best all-around preventive measure against pneumonia, not to mention hundreds of other illnesses, including many forms of cancer.

Other specific measures include having influenza and pneumonia vaccinations and taking 100 milligrams daily (under your doctor's supervision) of a drug called amantadine, which has been known to prevent type A influenza. Finally, if you have the flu, take it easy. Pneumonia can be the result of a flu that never went away because the person did not allow his or her body to mobilize all of its energies to fight the invader.

Several times you've mentioned pleurisy-like pain. What is pleurisy?

An inflammation of the pleura, which is the lining of the lung. The pain, as I've said, is sharp, often described as sandpaper rubbing against the inside of the chest. The pain can be agonizing at times. Often the pain is caused or made worse by the act of breathing, sometimes only by deep breathing, sometimes just by normal inhaling and exhaling. Frequently a cough or sneeze will make it worse. Sometimes *only* a cough or sneeze will make the chest hurt. It is even possible, though not so common, that movement, such as turning over in bed, can bring on—or make worse—the pain of pleurisy. And just as the brain may translate a stomach pain into a chest pain, so might the brain refer the pain of pleurisy to a different part of the body.

Why does the pleura become inflamed?

Bacteria, viruses, and parasites can cause an inflammation if they get into the body and reach the lining of the lungs. Tuberculosis can also cause pleurisy, as can any of the *collagen diseases* (connective tissue diseases) such as lupus. Even asbestos particles can cause this kind of inflammation if they get deep enough into the lungs to be deposited into the pleura. A collection of fluid in the lungs, known as pleural effusion, resulting from infections and other harmful agents, can swell up and stretch the pleura, causing an inflammation. Interestingly, although the fluid can cause pleurisy, it may also sometimes help ease the chest pain usually associated with this condition.

With any of these potential causes, the inflammation is usually located in one specific location on the lining of the lung and its onset is usually quite rapid.

How is a diagnosis made?

Because pleurisy pain can be the same as some heart attack pain or other cardiac conditions, such as *pericarditis* (an inflammation of the heart lining), these cardiac illnesses must first be ruled out with the appropriate investigative tools. Tumors of the wall of the chest and of the pleura can also cause pleurisy-like pain, and so these must also be watched for.

X rays often do not show pleurisy because such inflammation does not produce a shadow. Sometimes, however, the X rays will show fluid if there is any or adhesion (tissue stuck together and failing to move naturally). Sometimes the mediastinum (the middle of the chest) is actually pulled toward the inflamed area. Occasionally, a doctor can tell just by listening to your breathing or to your own description of symptoms that you have pleurisy.

How is pleurisy treated?

Because the pain is often excruciating, codeine and other painkillers are often necessary, as are cough suppressants if coughing is causing the pain to worsen.

Antibiotics are almost always employed against pleurisy because they counter bacteria—it's the most common cause—and keep the condition from leading to pneumonia. If the cause of pleurisy is tuberculosis, it must be treated accordingly. The treatment of pleurisy rarely will require hospitalization, but nevertheless you should take it seriously. If not treated, the pleura can rupture the adjacent lung tissue and can cause spontaneous *pneumothorax.*

What is spontaneous pneumothorax?

Pneumothorax is free air that gets into the pleural cavity—the area between the lining of the chest wall and the lining of the lung. This cavity is composed of a plastic wrap–like material that is supposed to allow the lungs to move up and down smoothly. Pneumothorax occurs when air leaks from the lungs into this chest region through a rupture in lung tissue. The resulting pain usually radiates right across the chest, but it can reach down into the abdomen or up into the shoulders. It is usually a sharp mid-chest pain associated with shortness of breath and may have an accompanying cough. You might hardly notice this condition at all or you might experience complete collapse and be unable to breathe.

PULMONARY-RELATED CHEST PAIN 61

The lung tissue just suddenly breaks open?

Yes. It can happen as the result of an asthma attack or an accident in which something pierces the chest, such as a fractured rib, a bullet, or a knife. It can result from an infected lung tissue, an abscess of lung tissue, tuberculosis, or from a sudden change in altitude (in high diving, for example).

What's the diagnosis and treatment?

Chest X rays will usually find the pneumothorax, although some smaller pneumothorax will only appear on an X ray if it is taken while you exhale. The smaller amounts of air in this region often require no more than medical observation to make sure that they don't enlarge. In most cases, the amount of leaked air is sufficiently small so that it can be absorbed relatively quickly. The gap responsible for the leak should heal on its own without complications. The leaked air of a larger pneumothorax can take up to four weeks to be absorbed. Sometimes there is so much air that it must be removed medically with a special vacuum device. The ruptured lung tissue should heal on its own, unless it is the result of an abscess, which may need to be removed, or pierced tissue, which may require surgical repair. If it is unhealthy lung tissue that may break open again, such tissue may need to be removed surgically before the rupture can heal.

Are there any other lung-related causes of chest pain?

There are a variety of chemicals that, when inhaled (sometimes even at minimal exposure), can cause chest pain and eventually cause lung disease. These include insecticides; various industrial gases; aerosols; the oxides of copper, iron, zinc, mercury; hydrocarbons such as gasoline, benzene, and other petroleum derivatives; burning oils, wood, and paper; sulphur dioxide; natural fungi; and organic dusts.

There are, in fact, pulmonary illnesses named specifically for the kinds of work environments that most often provoke them: Farmer's lung (caused by certain natural fungi), Bird Breeder's lung (caused by the inhalation of feather particles), Cheese Worker's lung (from mold and fungi), Paprika Splitter's lung (from dust and powder), Mushroom Worker's lung (from spores), Wood Pulp Worker's lung, and Coal Miner's lung, to name a few.

But if I don't work in any of these industries, do I have to worry about any of these illnesses?

Probably not, although you do need to be concerned about exposure to a dirty humidifier or air conditioner. These devices need to be cleaned regularly, and failure to do so can result in dust build-up and mold growth. A common mold growing on the air conditioners of America is Aspergillus, which is also responsible for athlete's foot. Exposure to any of these substances can cause chest pain and eventual lung disease. So can exposure to radiation.

Radiation? How would I be exposed to radiation in my everyday life?

Probably your greatest risk would be radon gas beneath your house. There has been much recent talk about the respiratory hazards of this gas and the relative ease with which it can be tested for and removed from your home. But that, unfortunately, is not all.

What else should I be cautious about to promote healthy lungs and to prevent chest pain?

Some prescription medicines have been known to cause inflammation of the lungs. If located near nerve endings, such inflammation can result in chest pain. It is not inconceivable that the side effect of *any* medicine could cause pulmonary-related chest pain in any given person. Those medications actually *reported* to have rendered such side effects in some people include the oral antidiabetic medicines tolbutamide and chlorpropamide, and heart medicines known as beta blockers (which, ironically, are sometimes used to help relieve cardiac chest pain). Even the very antibiotics used to treat many lung illnesses can themselves be the cause of pulmonary chest pain, as can some tranquilizers, antidepressants, and some cancer therapy drugs.

What can I do to protect myself?

Make sure you and your doctor closely monitor the use of any medicine and replace it if such side effects occur.

Are there any other causes of lung inflammation?

Rheumatoid arthritis, other connective tissue diseases, and blood vessel disorders may also cause pulmonary chest pain. Even chronic hepatitis (a disease of the liver) can inflame tissue above the liver at the base of the lung (just above the diaphragm), causing chest pain. Ulcerative colitis (of the colon) and ileitis (of the small intestines) can be associated with inflammation of the lung. These conditions are usually treatable if you simply tell your doctor about your chest pain and get started on the diagnostic trail.

There are also a host of not-yet-fully-understood lung inflammations and other disorders that are simply labeled as *idiopathic* (which means the doctor does not know the cause), such as idiopathic pulmonary inflammation and idiopathic pulmonary fibrosis.

How does a doctor treat a condition he or she doesn't yet fully understand?

As best he or she can at the given time with what is available. To begin with, the pain can be relieved using analgesic medications, cortisone drugs and dilating agents can restore normal breathing, and moisturizing agents can also be used. Sometimes a doctor has to experiment a little —using common sense and a pragmatic approach—before finding a therapy to which a given pulmonary chest pain will respond.

As with any known or unknown illness, there is always the possibility of an underlying cancer. In the case of pulmonary diseases, leukemia and lymphoma (tumor of the lymphatic system) must always be considered and ruled out if possible. Then, of course, there is always the unfortunate possibility that a chest pain can result from lung cancer.

I thought there might be something you were postponing.

I don't think anyone likes to think about lung cancer, and I can hardly blame them. But be reassured that if you don't smoke and you don't work in an environment that puts you in daily contact with toxic dust particles, your chances of ever being afflicted with lung cancer are lessened. Probably about 80%, give or take, of all lung cancer patients are cigarette smokers. If you do smoke or work in a polluted environment and quit (the cigarettes and/or the job or get your boss to clean up your air), then you may greatly reduce your lung cancer risk over a period of time.

Having said all that, I should emphasize that lung cancer is treatable, but recovery is rarely total. It is difficult to generalize, however, since there are a variety of different kinds of tumors that can appear on any part of the lung.

Are there any causes other than smoking and inhaling industrial dust?

It is possible that metastatic cancer, which is cancer that has spread from another part of the body, can settle on the lung. I want to reemphasize the potential effects of the environment here. We don't yet fully understand the long-term effects of air pollution. That's why it's important to know the quality of your air and respond accordingly. It's not a bad idea for all of us to try and improve what has become a pretty shameful situation in the skies of our cities.

As for the unknown number of unknown causes of cancer —any kind of cancer, including lung cancer—these account for only a small minority of cases.

What kind of chest pain are we talking about?

There is no specific kind of pain that tells a doctor that this man or that woman has lung cancer. The pain is often determined by the location of the cancer on the lung and can be of virtually any kind I have described. It can be intense or mild or barely noticeable (probably the worst kind since it is the least likely to instigate an early diagnosis). The chest pain can be accompanied by shortness of breath, fever, pneumonia, bronchitis, hoarseness, weight loss, and back pain. Coughing is almost always a symptom of lung cancer, sometimes with a bloody sputum.

How is lung cancer treated?

The removal of lung tissue is a possibility if the cancer has not spread outside its fibrous sac. In the latter case, a large surrounding area of tissue may be removed along with up to about 40% of the lung volume. This kind of radical surgery is performed in an attempt to remove the cancer entirely from the body so that there is no chance of its spreading.

Very rarely will a surgeon remove one of the two lungs in an attempt to halt any cancerous migration. Other treatments include chemotherapy and radiation therapy to try and contain the cancer.

There are also some more controversial approaches to this as well as other cancers. These include therapies allied to nutritional findings. There is, for example, a theory associating *free radicals* (broken bits of molecules missing an electron) in the body with cancer. Antioxidants, such as betacarotene and vitamin C, seem to neutralize these free radicals. Linus Pauling, for this and other reasons, has been asserting for years that megadosing with vitamin C can reduce the cancer risk and possibly help treat cancer once it occurs. Another nutritional aid against cancer are the cruciferous vegetables, those of the cabbage family, which contain substances that seem to have detoxification qualities.

Other speculative techniques thought possibly to prevent the onset or spread of cancer are visualization, subliminal tapes, and other mental and emotional therapies. Although there are no statistics to support the claims of any of these methods of treatment, it is becoming increasingly clear that emotions and attitudes do play a significant role in the treatment of any illness, especially cancer. The mind, when used in tandem with medicine, is a powerful tool. Use it.

Mediastinal Chest Pain

What's a mediastinum and what's it supposed to do?

The *mediastinum* is the space between the lungs and the heart. It is, in medical terms, divided into three parts. The front of the mediastinum—the part closest to the *sternum* (breastbone) and underneath it—contains the thymus gland, which manufactures immune cells.

What are the other parts of the mediastinum?

The middle section houses lymph nodes, the aorta, and the heart. Lymph nodes are part of the immune system, comprising a filter system for removing bacteria and other invaders from the lungs. The aorta is the large artery leaving the heart and delivering blood throughout the body. A significant segment of the aorta passes through the mediastinum. The rear of the mediastinum, also known as the *posterium,* contains nerve tissue and major blood vessels.

And what causes chest pain in the mediastinum?

For starters, a fracture of the sternum or a tumor of the thymus gland can render the front mediastinum very painful. In the middle area, lymph node enlargement in reaction to infection, leukemia, lymphomas, and sarcoid can all cause chest pain.

Sarcoid? Is that a kind of cancer?

No one is quite sure. The cause of this illness remains the subject of much debate, though some suspect it may be viral in nature or result from immune system abnormalities. There may also be a genetic predisposition. It resembles tuberculosis and, like tuberculosis, it forms lung nodules called granulomas, but it is a distinctly different disease. It can cause a variety of symptoms, including chest pain, which should be reported immediately to your physician so that he or she can rule out sarcoid or discover it early and begin treatment with cortisone.

Any other middle-area causes of chest pain?

Probably the most serious condition of this area of the mediastinum—and it is a very serious condition—would be a dissecting aortic aneurism.

What's an aortic aneurism?

Any abnormal dilation in any specific part of the aorta. Even though aortic aneurisms are relatively uncommon, when they do occur, it is often in the mediastinal area.

Why would it become dilated?

No one is really sure. It is believed to be a somewhat rare genetic defect.

Why does the aortic aneurism dissect?

The abnormal dilation causes a stretching, a ballooning out, and a weakening of the ballooned aortic tissue. It can even weaken to the point of rupturing spontaneously, although a rupture from the eventual dissection (the peeling apart of layers of tissue) is a greater, and much more likely, concern.

How does that happen?

Plaque—the infamous sludge of cholesterol—builds up in the already-weakened tissue of the aortic aneurism. Blood seeps into the walls of the aneurism, like water seeping between the layers of an onion, and dissects those layers, peeling them apart. Ultimately, it can peel the whole aortic wall apart and destroy it, causing an aortic rupture with severe internal hemorrhaging.

When it ruptures, what kind of chest pain does it cause?

I have heard it described as exquisite, incredible, sharp, tearing, constant, unrelenting, and "living hell." One patient of mine said he felt as if he were being ripped in two. This was not surprising since the most important blood vessel in his entire body had just been torn.

If the pain strikes in the front part of the chest, it usually means the dissection is going upward toward the heart. The pain often goes from the center of the chest right through to the back, the neck, or down into the stomach. If the pain hits in the mid or upper back, the dissection is probably on the left extension of the aorta. Other back pain can result if the dissecting aneurism is located on the part of the aorta passing through the abdomen.

These guidelines are not always correct, but they underscore the importance of communicating your exact pain experience to your doctor so that he or she can diagnose and treat this condition. Other accompanying symptoms can include a cough and shortness of breath and possibly incapacitation. A dissecting aortic aneurism is commonly mistaken for a severe heart attack—and it is no less serious.

Is it always caused by atherosclerosis?

Usually. It can also be the result of hypertension and even a long-term complication of syphilis.

What's the treatment?

Surgery. That means call the paramedics. Dissecting aortic aneurism is a medical emergency. Diagnosis can be made with X rays, though they are not the most reliable. Dye studies, called aortography, are not always effective either. Ultrasound can usually make an accurate diagnosis if the dissection is in the abdominal area. In the chest area, however, too much air can reduce the soundwave picture. The most precise diagnosis is made with a CT or MRI (magnetic resonance imaging) scan, but, because this requires time and there may not be any, diagnosis must often be made on the operating table.

What kind of operation is done?

A graft of skin is attached to the torn section of the aorta or the aorta is completely replaced with an artificial one. These procedures are often successful if performed in time.

Anything in particular I should do to make sure this never happens to me?

There are no guarantees but, if you follow my guidelines for the prevention of heart disease, you may reduce the risk of this and many other conditions. If you have any reason to believe you might be at risk, have your doctor examine your aorta as part of your regular checkup. And, if you ever get syphilis, treat it immediately.

You said it was a rare problem. How rare?

In my own practice, I'd say I encounter one about every four years. If everyone maintained low cholesterol and blood pressure, I might never have to treat another one.

How about chest pain from the posterium?

In the posterium of the mediastinum, pain can be caused by thoracic spine disease such as disc degeneration, spinal tumors, or spine fractures, blood vessel abnormalities, and tumors of the nerve tissue.

What kind of pain are we talking about?

Nothing specific. These conditions can cause any kind of chest pain and therefore they are likely to be diagnosed only after your doctor has ruled out many other possible causes of chest pain. Diagnosis may be a lengthy process, and it is important for the patient not to believe that because no cause is found, no cause exists. Some of these mediastinum conditions are, like most other causes of chest pain, potentially quite serious, and the severity—or lack of severity—of the pain may have no relation to the seriousness of the condition. So, don't hesitate in responding to a chest pain and encourage your doctor's persistence in reaching a diagnosis.

What about treatment?

As with any tumors, early detection and treatment is crucial and can be life-saving. This is no less true in the posterium or any part of the mediastinum. In fact most causes of mediastinal chest pain are treatable if the pain is reported immediately to your doctor so that he or she can make a diagnosis.

Chest Wall Pain

What exactly is my chest wall? Are we talking about ribs?

Yes, and we're also talking about the skin, muscles, tissue, and nerves that compose the organic barrier protecting your upper internal organs.

How might the chest wall cause chest pain?

A common chest wall pain syndrome is called intercostal neuritis. That's an inflammation of the nerves around the chest wall and often in and around the sternum area. These nerves run from the spinal cord to the chest wall area right between the ribs, hence the name intercostal neuritis. *Intercostal* means between the ribs, *neuritis* is an inflammation of a nerve or nerves. These nerves can be inflamed by a virus of any kind, even the herpes virus, which decides—and viruses are quite capricious by nature—to settle in the intercostal nerves. Often, in the case of herpes, a doctor may have difficulty in making a diagnosis until herpes lesions are visible on the surface of the skin served by these nerves.

And this causes a chest pain?

Yes. In fact, intercostal neuritis pain is frequently confused with heart attack pain. The pain is often sharp and lacerating, like a knife plunged into the chest. It is usually described as excessive, intense, and debilitating. It can, however, also be felt as the sandpaper-rubbing pain of pleurisy. The pain can sometimes feel like an electric shock. Sometimes the pain will even disappear, along with any and all other sensation in that particular chest area.

One quality of this particular pain that usually differentiates it from a heart attack is that it is usually brought on or made worse by movements, such as jumping, sneezing, or even the strain of defecation. If the patient is able to hold completely still, the pain of intercostal neuritis will usually subside temporarily.

One quality of the pain of intercostal neuritis that usually differs from that of pleurisy is that breathing tends *not* to bring on or exacerbate this particular pain.

What's the treatment?

There is no specific treatment other than to treat the virus that may have caused the condition if it is still present. If it is an opportunistic virus, as is usually the case with herpes, you may be immune-suppressed and need to modify your nutrition and lifestyle to strengthen your immunity. Opportunistic viral causes of intercostal neuritis may also be symptomatic of an underlying malignancy, and so you should communicate with your doctor about your pain right away.

The intercostal neuritis itself is a condition that the body will recover from on its own. Your overall health will probably affect your body's ability to heal this inflammation, though this has not been proven. The most important thing you can do, with regard to intercostal neuritis, is to have it properly diagnosed and don't allow yourself, if you ever get another chest pain, to assume that it is a recurrence of this particular condition.

Another illness that can be serious in the same way —in that it can feel like a heart attack and later make a heart attack feel like *it*—is called *costochondritis*.

And what is that?

It's an inflammation of the *costal cartilages,* which attach the ribs to the sternum. Usually it involves the third or fourth rib; thus, its location is directly in front of the heart. In some rare cases there are reddened areas above these cartilage attachments, which is known as Tietze's syndrome.

What causes this inflammation?

A virus, bacteria, arthritis, or any number of unknowns.

And you say this causes pain much like that of a heart attack?

Because of its location, the pain of costochondritis is probably the most easily mistaken for a heart attack. It can be a dull, achy pain or a sharp, piercing pain. The pain is almost always felt right in the mid-chest area, exactly where the inflammation has occurred. It is usually described as being worse when lying down, worse at night, though not at all made worse by breathing. It can be dull and tolerable or it can be unbearable.

How does a doctor know that it's not a heart attack?

There is actually a very simple diagnostic technique. By finding the space between rib, cartilage, and sternum and by applying pressure, a doctor can usually tell if what you have is costochondritis. If it is, the pain will get much worse from the pressure. However, your doctor may still take an EKG to make sure you're not suffering from costochondritis *and* a heart attack at the same time.

CHEST WALL PAIN 75

What is the treatment for costochondritis?

Your doctor will likely prescribe ice packs, analgesic as well as antiarthritic medications, and other nonsteroidal antiinflammatory drugs (*nonsteroidal* indicates, specifically, any antiinflammatory other than cortisone).

Are there any significant dangers of nontreatment of costochondritis?

Pain, pain, and more pain. As for other physical complications, I have not encountered any in my practice. I would say it is more than likely that the inflammation will heal on its own. I would even guess that some very masochistic people often go without ever having it diagnosed. But that doesn't completely rule out the possibility of complications. The inflammation could, conceivably, spread to the *pericardium,* which is the lining of the heart itself.

Are there any other causes of chest wall pain?

Yes. There are a number of known and probably a great many unknown causes. Arthritis can afflict joints, bones, and/or cartilage—not just in the wrists and ankles but anywhere in the skeleton, including the ribs, sternum, and rib attachments—and thus can cause a chest pain. Such pain can result from any of the hundreds of strains of arthritis, including lupus arthritis and rheumatoid arthritis, an autoimmune disorder (an illness in which, for unknown reasons, the immune system turns on itself). The arthritis can also afflict the muscle and tendon attachments in the chest wall, which is a condition called fibromyositis. Arthritis that attacks the spine is known as spondylitis and is likely to cause back pain but can also cause chest pain.

What is the treatment for arthritic chest pain?

The treatment of arthritis remains varied. No one can come to any consensus on *one* correct method, and arthritic conditions that cause chest pain are no exception. There are at least 120 different diseases that fall under the diagnosis of arthritis, and entire books attempt to offer insight into the treatment of this still-elusive disease. I can, however, offer some basic recommendations.

There are many medications used for both pain relief and treatment of arthritis. Effective chemical therapy depends on accurate diagnosis of the arthritis. Antiinflammatory drugs, for example, are not likely to be effective in treating noninflammatory arthritis. Treatment depends to some degree on which of the three general types of arthritis is at play.

The first type, noninflammatory arthritis, results from degeneration of cartilage at the edge of bones. This can occur from abuse-related degeneration, the trauma of an injury, or just regular wear and tear. Osteoarthritis is a common type of noninflammatory arthritis. Inflammatory arthritis, the second type, is probably the most common. It is most often caused by cell and membrane damage from autoimmune chemicals, stress, or food allergies. Inflammatory arthritis involves bones, muscles, tendons, or connective tissue. The third general type of arthritis is infectious arthritis, resulting from bacterial or viral infections in the joints.

If an arthritic chest pain is the result of a food allergy, treatment begins with determining the allergy and ceasing exposure to the particular food or food group.

In virtually all types of arthritis, cigarette smoking and the consumption of coffee, alcohol, excess salt, citrus fruits, refined sugars, and refined carbohydrates can often exacerbate the condition, as will tension, anger, and other negative stress emotions.

A diet built around fresh vegetables and non-citrus fruits, fresh deep-water fish, nonfat dairy products, twelve to fourteen glasses of purified water each day, and an ambitious vitamin and mineral supplement program (described later) is very helpful in combating arthritis, especially arthritis caused by autoimmune disease.

The medical establishment has yet to fully embrace any of these recommendations, but, since they all conform to a lifestyle that reduces the risk of many other illnesses, including heart disease, there is no reason to wait for FDA approval.

Exercise is also an important part of the treatment of arthritis. I have seen countless patients of mine reduce their arthritic pain drastically in all parts of their bodies, including the chest area, by walking, by doing hatha-yoga, or by exercising in swimming pools.

Of course, before you start engaging in aquatic aerobics, have your doctor make sure your supposedly arthritic rib is not in fact a rib fracture. The two conditions can produce similar chest pains.

Wouldn't I know it if I had fractured a rib?

Not necessarily. Every year doctors see countless cases of people who've had a little too much to drink, swallow, smoke, or snort or who are on sedatives for medical reasons fall into a filing cabinet, a podium, or a subway turnstile without much awareness of what they're doing, and then awaken with an excruciating chest pain, believing it is a heart attack.

Those of us who abstain from alcohol and controlled substances and who generally behave in a manner that would not cause a doctor to want to sedate us need not worry about that sort of thing?

Not exactly. It is possible to fracture a rib while sneezing or coughing during a bout with the flu. Anyone with *osteoporosis,* whose bones are decalcified and brittle, can break a rib spontaneously from the slightest trauma and suffer a chest pain.

What kind of chest pain?

Any kind, really, from a dull ache in a local area to a knife-like sharp pain. Sometimes the pain is made worse by breathing or other movement.

What is the usual treatment for a fractured rib?

Your physician must first be sure the fracture is "in line," so that there is no chance any broken piece of rib can cut the lung tissue. An X ray can usually clear up that matter. After that, time and analgesics will work to heal the fracture.

Does that take care of the chest wall?

Yes. There is always the possibility of *bursitis* (an inflammation of a bursa, a lining that allows ligaments or tendons to move without friction), *myositis* (any muscle inflammation) in the chest wall muscles, or other muscle, bone, joint, cartilage, and tissue disease. There is also a syndrome called xiphodynia (pronounced zy-pho-din-ee-a), a sudden pain in the front of the chest associated with the *xiphoid process,* which is the very bottom tip of the sternum. This pain is usually felt deep in the chest and sometimes in the back. It is often made worse by eating a heavy meal or by motion, especially stooping. The pain is made much worse by rubbing the area and can last anywhere from ten minutes to ten days. Its cause is yet to be known, and so the treatment is most likely to avoid activities that make the pain worse until it goes away.

This and other little-known conditions are not, generally, life-threatening, except insofar as they can mask a heart attack.

Other Physical Noncardiac Conditions Known to Cause Chest Pain

Have we come to the miscellaneous, end-of-the-road noncardiac chest pain?

This is it, except for psychologically induced chest pain, which will follow this section.

Are you now going to tell us that, because of the proximity of our nerve circuitry within the body and within the brain, any illness anywhere in our bodies can be felt as a chest pain?

Not quite, though I cannot say that's not true. I've never heard of anyone twisting an ankle and getting a chest pain —with the exception perhaps of Mary Decker during the finals of the 1984 Olympics. I suppose anything is possible, but I can only refer to chest pain causation I have read about or observed. For example, arthritis in the neck or collarbone as well as any part of the spine can produce a chest pain.

Why is that?

I can only guess that it has to do with the reading of the nerve endings in the brain. For probably the same reason, bursitis in the shoulder can result in a chest pain. So can fibromyositis.

What is fibromyositis?

It's a musculoskeletal disease causing inflammation and swelling, usually of the neck, though it can also afflict the shoulders or any other muscle groups.

What kind of chest pain does it produce?

Usually a generalized ache in the upper chest. Sometimes, though, it can be pinpointed to tender spots between the second and third ribs. It is often reported to cause stiffness, fatigue, and sometimes insomnia.

What causes fibromyositis?

No one knows for sure. It could be caused by a virus, infection, gout, arthritis, trauma, immune system disease, food or other allergy, or an unknown cause.

What's the treatment?

Virtually the same as for arthritis. Sometimes cortisone is used along with heat applications and gentle massage. Stress reduction is important and that means patience with a healing process that will take time.

Anything else?

Have I mentioned back strain? It is possible to throw out your back and catch a pain in the chest. Or you can injure a disc and one of your symptoms—possibly the *only* symptom—might be a chest pain. An orthopedist I know even tells me that injuries or illnesses of the muscles in the back of the neck, the trapeziuses, the rhomboids, certain spinal muscles, the pectorals, and the biceps can all produce chest pain. Even poor posture can cause a chest pain.

I've heard of poor posture and back pain ... but chest pain?

Poor posture can cause an interior compression against nerve roots from the spine that serve the chest area. This kind of compression can cause chest pain. A recent example of this can be found in people working all day in front of video display terminals. The position of the chair, the hands, and the neck amounts to poor posture and may explain why these workers have a significant incidence of this kind of noncardiac chest pain.

How are these conditions treated?

In the case of poor posture, a more humanely designed desk and chair and more frequent work breaks may be the only prescription. As for more serious back and disc problems, a trip to the orthopedist may be in order. This underscores the importance of a timely and aggressive diagnosis of a chest pain.

Any other miscellaneous causes of chest pain?

Sickle-cell anemia, a genetic disorder most common in people of African descent, can cause chest pain.

82 NONCARDIAC CAUSES OF CHEST PAIN

What exactly is sickle-cell anemia?

It's a disease of red blood cells resulting in *hemolysis* (cell wall breakage); the cells become misshapen and resemble sickles.

What kind of chest pain can this cause?

Usually acute sharp chest pain, muscle pain, and/or joint pain. It can be accompanied by abdominal pain, back pain, frequent vomiting, shortness of breath, lung degeneration, and enlarged heart.

Is there any treatment?

Unfortunately, there isn't much. Sickle-cell anemia remains a disease without a cure. Sometimes a *splenectomy* is performed (surgical removal of the spleen) in an attempt to stop more and more red blood cells from becoming sickle cells.

Does that cover all the miscellaneous causes of chest pain?

Not quite. High blood pressure, though known as the silent killer, can occasionally cause a chest pain. There is no clearly prevailing medical theory as to why the silent killer will sometimes speak up, but when it does it can be a blessing. Hypertension (which we will discuss in more detail in the coronary prevention section) can usually be dealt with medically. If untreated, it can be a major contributing factor to heart disease, just like another miscellaneous cause of chest pain known as *hyperthyroidism.*

What's hyperthyroidism?

It's a fancy way of describing an overactive thyroid gland that produces excess hormones. The instigator of this condition is still under debate, but it is becoming increasingly clear that hyperthyroidism is *not* a disease exclusively of young people. In people over 40 it is often preceded by a major bout with stress. It is yet to be established whether the stress causes the overactive thyroid gland or whether the excess hormones produced might be causing the stress. The symptoms of hyperthyroidism are wide-ranging. They include fatigue, weakness, irritability, anxiety, insomnia, mood swings, intolerance to heat, rapid pulse, heart irregularities, high blood pressure, shortness of breath, and any of the different types of chest pain.

Is it treatable?

Most doctors use isotope or prescriptive therapy. Caffeine, alcohol, and tobacco must be eliminated from the diet, which is not a bad idea anyway even if you don't suffer from hyperthyroidism, because these drugs are all known to cause chest pain.

Smoking a cigarette or drinking too much coffee makes your chest hurt?

It can. So can snorting cocaine. The use and abuse of these drugs can cause a noncardiac chest pain, and they can also, we all know, cause a heart attack. *Amphetamines* (central nervous system stimulant drugs) can also cause chest pain and, when used in excess, can increase the risk of heart disease.

Is there any specific kind of chest pain?

Not really. These drugs can result in any of the kinds of chest pain I have described, including chest pain that feels just like a heart attack.

And the treatment?

Stop using cocaine, caffeine, and amphetamines (uppers), and quit smoking. If you don't, then you'd better memorize the second half of this book, because you are putting yourself at serious risk for heart disease. I know that quitting is easier said than done. It may also be easier than recovering from a heart attack.

Since this is a survival guide for a heart attack, any tips on kicking these dangerous habits?

I can tell you that a recent study published in the *Journal of the American Medical Association* found that, regardless of the overall quit-smoking method—and there are many, from acupuncture to nicotine chewing gum—the one single factor that most helped smokers quit was human contact. Smokers who had the most frequent face-to-face contact with a counselor or other supporting person developed the most long-lasting motivation to stay away from the weed. This should come as no surprise to anyone. I would suspect it is true for any habit or addiction. As for cigarettes in particular, there is a high blood pressure drug called clonidine that preliminary research has found to help ease nicotine cravings. You may want to ask your doctor about it. As for caffeine, it is not a good idea to quit cold turkey because the withdrawals from this drug can be quite serious. A gradual reduction to complete elimination is the best approach.

Psychological Causes of Chest Pain

We have all felt a sudden fright right in our chest, and a broken heart sometimes feels like a broken heart, but can psychologically induced chest pain really get so bad that it can be mistaken for a heart attack?

Absolutely. Emotional stresses and other activities of the mind can precipitate a vast number of conditions within the body, including chest pain that feels exactly like a heart attack.

There now exists an enormous body of evidence to support the mind-body/body-mind connection. A very recent study involving multiple personalities produced startling results. A man had several personalities, none of them consciously aware of the others. All but one of these personalities was allergic to orange juice. The one personality that was not allergic was the personality of a child who loved orange juice. Researchers discovered that, if the man while in the personality of the child began to drink orange juice and then assumed another personality, he broke out in hives. Yet, if he reverted to being the child personality, the hives went away. With cases like this before us, words like *psychosomatic* (which means a disorder caused by or notably influenced by the emotional state of the patient) become superfluous.

Almost *any* disorder is affected by the mental state of the patient, just as almost any disorder affects the mental state of the patient. Some conditions are probably more directly connected to mental and emotional activities. Immune suppression and cancer seem most often to fall into this category. So does chest pain.

Are you saying that the mind plays a role in causing physical conditions, which in turn cause chest pain?

That is part of what I am saying. Yes, almost any of the conditions I have described thus far can be brought on or be made worse by anxiety, depression, anger, fear, panic, guilt, and other negative emotions. Esophageal spasms, for example, can result from acute anxiety that upsets the autonomic nervous system.

But there are also a great many cases in which the patient describes a chest pain that sounds very much like heart disease—and not only is the heart in good shape but also the doctor can find no other organic cause for the described pain. I have seen this phenomenon countless times in my practice and a recent study done at the Veterans Administration Medical Center in Syracuse, New York, has confirmed my long-time suspicion. This study found that 30% of all patients with chest pain had nothing physically wrong with them. There are not many concrete facts with regard to this phenomenon. Doctors simply understand that a chest pain, like a headache, can be a symptom of emotional tension. Often the patient does not know to what he or she might be reacting. He or she does not simply say, "Oh, yes, I was fired from my job, my mother had a stroke, and my dog got hit by a car. . . . " or, "I'm afraid to be alone . . . , I'm afraid of the cold . . . , I'm afraid to leave the house, afraid to even take a shower."

Sometimes the instigating emotion is being suppressed consciously or unconsciously and, in a sense, is triggering a chest pain as a cry for help. Sometimes a chest pain might be a delayed reaction to last night's anger, last week's stress, or last month's panic or depression.

Is any one emotion more likely to trigger this reaction than any other?

Probably. Though, as with most questions you could ask about this kind of chest pain, there are no empirical facts. My guess would be that panic disorder, which has been written about extensively as an autonomous cause of chest pain, is the most prevalent.

What exactly is panic disorder?

It is a growing epidemic in modern American life, beginning with panic attacks, which are intense and often debilitating bouts of fear, anxiety, terror, and other similar emotions that seem to come from nowhere. Such attacks are reported in ever-increasing and alarming numbers all over the country (and probably throughout much of the rest of the world). Most people, at some time in their lives, experience a panic attack. A one-time panic attack or even a once-in-a-while attack may be considered one of the normal hazards of modern life. If these attacks occur more than four times within a four-week period or if a panic attack is followed by a persistent fear of another attack, most psychiatrists would probably agree that they were dealing with a case of panic disorder, which, if not dealt with, can create a serious threat to good health and the ability to function.

Are there any other symptoms that might help me know if I'm having a panic attack?

Well, I wouldn't necessarily want anyone to make that diagnosis on his or her own. There are a number of symptoms doctors use in determining whether a patient has had one or more panic attacks. These symptoms, as defined by the

American Psychiatric Association, are shortness of breath (sometimes hyperventilation and a sense of smothering, sometimes a sense of choking), sweating, dizziness, unsteadiness, nausea, gastrointestinal distress, numbness or tingling in the fingers or other bodily extremities, hot or chilly flashes, shaking, tremors, fear (not surprisingly) of losing control, fear of death, fear of insanity (even fear of fear), tachycardia (rapid heart rate), other irregular heart rhythms, and, of course, chest pain.

What kind of chest pain are we talking about?

Virtually any kind, from sharp to dull, specific to general, tolerable to excruciating. More often than not, the pain is like that of a coronary: substernal pain or belt-like mid-chest pain, intense, often radiating to the neck, jaw, and wrist areas, possibly compressive, possibly sharp, and with an associated feeling of impending doom. In these cases, the triggering emotion may actually be fear of a heart attack so that, as the chest pain begins to come on, the fear intensifies, which intensifies the pain. These people may have lost one or both parents or another close relative to heart disease. Often these people know much about heart disease; their descriptions of their symptoms sometimes sound like accurate paraphrasings of a medical text. This is not to say that they are faking. They are not. The pain is real.

Is there any physiological explanation of how a mental process causes an actual physical pain?

Medical researchers are no longer so certain that a mental process is not, at the same time, a physical process. As for specific explanations, there is much speculation, all still controversial. It is possible, for example, that panic disorder —especially when precipitated by anxiety connected with fear of heart disease—can, for whatever reason, cause spasms in the intercostal chest wall area. These spasms may explain the resulting chest pain.

Not so controversial is the reason why anxiety and panic can speed up or cause irregularities in heart rhythms. The theory is that the body, under a certain amount of adverse stress, seems to release what are called "fight-or-flight" chemicals (adrenal-like chemicals that ready the body to either defend its life or run for its life). Although most of us do not encounter situations regularly in our daily lives in which fight or flight is necessary, our bodies have not evolved to be able to differentiate the fears of contemporary life—often non-life-threatening ones, like fear of intimacy, fear of failure, or fear of success. We might react, therefore, to rumors of layoffs in our workplace much as an ancestor of 10,000 years ago might have reacted to confrontation with a bear. What we don't yet know but may one day discover is that these fight-or-flight chemicals released by anxiety and panic are biochemically causing this unexplained chest pain.

For now we do know that the hyperventilation associated with panic attacks can, by itself, cause pain in any part of the chest simply by the sheer strain it puts on those muscles.

If the mind-body connection is such a close link, can a physical factor be the cause of a panic disorder?

Absolutely. Panic disorders are not always completely emotional in nature. There are a number of physical illnesses now believed to precipitate panic disorder in some people. A tumor of the adrenal gland, for example, might release excess adrenaline and instigate a panic attack, which in turn might cause a chest pain. Panic attacks can also be symptomatic of asthma, lung obstruction, infection, hyperthyroidism, heart irregularities, and drug withdrawal in people who quit cold turkey from an addiction to Valium or amphetamine. Nutritional deficiencies, as well as food and other allergies, are also a common cause of panic disorder. A common deficiency causing panic attacks is lack of body calcium. An example of a food allergy is a gluten allergy (an allergy to wheat and wheat products). There are people for whom eating one slice of bread can make them completely irrational and incapacitated, often with accompanying chest pain.

What's the treatment for panic disorder?

Treatment is varied and often in-depth, although no one has come up with one surefire cure.

Certainly, if you have an allergy to gluten or some other food or substance, diagnosis and strict avoidance of the allergen may be all that is necessary. Deficiencies can often be corrected by dietary changes and supplementation. If there is an underlying physical illness, it must be treated.

Otherwise, some kind of psychiatric intervention may be required (though, interestingly, most panic disorder patients make their first visit to a regular physician). Sometimes a prior trauma—like a rape or combat in a war—must be dealt with. About 60% of all panic disorders can be resolved successfully through psychotherapy. Sometimes chemical therapies are needed. Some drugs commonly used under the supervision of physicians or psychotherapists in order to treat panic disorder are imipramine, beta blockers, and alprazolam.

I would never hesitate to recommend hatha-yoga or any other relaxation and breathing techniques at any stage of treatment. Knowing how to relax and deep breathe can help relieve hyperventilation and other symptoms, including chest pain before it becomes acute, should anxiety or panic attack recur. Very often, what can happen to people who possess no relaxation skills is that hyperventilation and the inability to get a good breath can make them panic even more and try desperately to draw in more air, often by raising their shoulders, which actually *restricts* the amount of air the lungs can hold and increases the pain, further exacerbating the panic attack.

It sounds like not treating panic disorder can be dangerous.

That's quite an understatement. As I've said with respect to other cases, the chest pain of a panic attack can be a blessing. It can save your life not only because it can be a symptom of a serious illness but also because if not dealt with medically the stress and tension can greatly increase the risk of heart disease and probably increase the risk of cancer over time. In the short run it often leads to a sense of doom—sometimes even suicidal urges—and it can easily be the acorn from which the tree of agoraphobia may grow.

Agoraphobia?

That's an acute fear of leaving one's house or immediate environment. A person stricken with frequent panic attacks will often begin to avoid places he or she suspects are triggers for such attacks. Soon any place can begin to have this effect, and thus the person is afraid to go anywhere.

Panic attacks, whether or not they're related to agoraphobia, can also be followed by bouts of severe depression, another potential cause of chest pain.

Depression causes chest pain?

The medical profession is still working on theories as to why this is, but my guess at this point would be that depression causes chest pain in many people for the same reason orange juice makes that gentleman with the multiple personalities break out in hives when he changes personalities in the middle of his breakfast. Most of us, no matter how scientific our background, grow up with some belief that the heart is the center of emotion—no matter how definitively we are taught in school that this is not true. Perhaps being conditioned to regard the pain of rejection or loss as a broken heart causes us to experience real chest pain when stricken with that kind of depression. But that raises the question of how we came to associate our emotional center with the heart muscle. Was it a fluke? Or is there some biochemical connection between the emotional processes of the brain and the pain nerves in heart muscle cells? I wonder whether some of our mammal cousins feel sadness in their chest.

In any case, the most important thing is to understand that depression can cause severe chest pain, which is another reason to take prolonged or acute depression seriously as a physical as well as an emotional illness.

What is the treatment for depression?

Entire books try to answer that question. It's a huge subject, in part because there are so many potential known and unknown causes of depression. In order to treat depression, you have to know whether the problem is a biochemical imbalance in the brain or the death of a loved one or a reaction to a food allergy or the aftereffects of extreme anxiety. In some cases, we treat the depression by treating its cause. But sometimes—as in the case of a death—we can't. Sometimes psychotherapy can help. Sometimes all we need to do is change our diet. In cases of acute depression, antidepressant drugs are often warranted (their potential side effects are less threatening than this sometimes paralyzing disease). If you are mildly depressed, vigorous walking and other exercise can do wonders for the depression and its resulting chest pain. Exercise releases natural antidepressant chemicals in the body known as endorphins, which elevate serotonin, a neurotransmitter (message carrier) in the brain that seems to calm us. But, of course, this must be done under a doctor's supervision. Unless you've established that a chest pain is *not* cardiac, a vigorous walk may be a suicide mission.

You say that people with a history of heart disease in their family often suffer chest pain of psychological origins. Are any other groups at a particularly high risk?

Yes. Those with a history of heart disease are probably not the most likely victims of emotionally rooted chest pain, though many of them also fall into the group that is most at risk. According to the most recent studies, this group seems to be people with type A personalities.

What is a type A personality?

I call them victims of "hurry-up disease" because they are stereotypically always in a hurry, seemingly in a hurry to do things, to accomplish, though in reality they may very well be hurrying up their own death. Common symptoms of the type A personality are obsessiveness, compulsiveness, impatience, and anger. They are often cynics, often perfectionists. These people may be successful in their professional lives—sometimes they achieve more superficial success in their personal lives—but they are rarely, if ever, satisfied. Not surprisingly, they tend to be well-educated, and there are many professions, such as lawyer, stockbroker, brain surgeon, motion picture director, politician, or political consultant, that can make such intense demands on an individual that in some cases it takes an extremely concerted effort not to become stricken with hurry-up disease and all of its complications. Medical schools, law schools, engineering schools, and aviation schools don't teach courses in relaxation and patience. Men under 40 seem to be most at risk, although women are quickly catching up. It may be, though this is only speculation, that the reason estimates of type A behavior and panic disorder curve downward after 40 is that the illness may be taking its toll in heart attacks and other illnesses—or at least scaring some people into a new lifestyle and a new outlook on life.

Heart attacks?

That's right. Not only can panic disorder and depression, if not dealt with, increase the risk of heart disease and other illnesses, but also the fact is that even if type A behavior does *not* cause panic attacks or depression, those people with hurry-up disease are still among the most likely to have a coronary.

So not only are they the most likely to have a psychologically induced chest pain and think they're having a heart attack, but they are also the most likely actually to be having a heart attack.

What can a person do to overcome hurry-up disease?

Slow down. Give up that perpetual struggle to control everything around you in your effort to regain control of your own mind and body. In many cases psychotherapy is the best approach. Since that is not my field I can offer no details; I can tell you, however, that I have seen results in my own patients who have dealt with their hurry-up disease either with a therapist or in group therapy. I can also tell you that pursuing meaningful human relationships can certainly change your lifestyle and possibly help curb stress. Taking the time to read a book or listen to Mozart can do wonders, at least in the short term. Learning to laugh, to trust someone or something, and to make compromises are also great steps toward recovery.

Part Two
WHEN YOUR HEART SPEAKS, LISTEN!

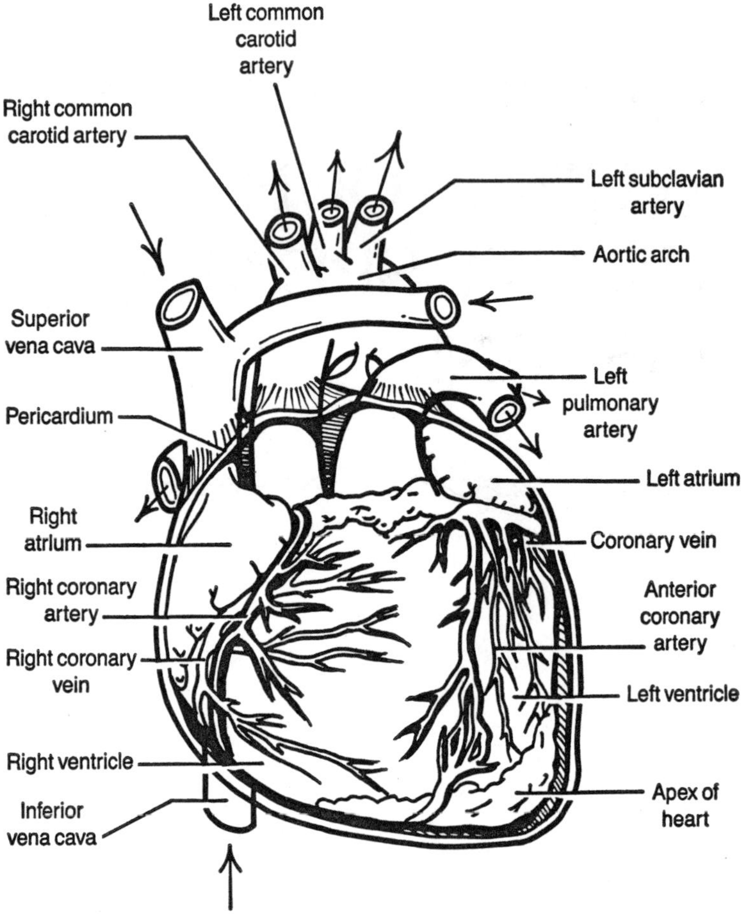

Left common carotid artery
Right common carotid artery
Left subclavian artery
Aortic arch
Superior vena cava
Left pulmonary artery
Pericardium
Left atrium
Right atrium
Coronary vein
Right coronary artery
Anterior coronary artery
Right coronary vein
Left ventricle
Right ventricle
Apex of heart
Inferior vena cava

FIGURE 2

A heartbeat is probably the first sound any of us hears as we float in the placenta, waiting to join the world. It is the sound that a fetus projects to let us know he or she is alive and well. It is the sound of life itself—and quite likely the root of all musical expression. It is also the sound of about 100,000 contractions pumping as much as 2,000 gallons of blood per day through the circulatory system.

The heart itself (figure 2) is a muscular organ composed of four chambers: two sides, right and left, each with a ventricle and an atrium. Blood is pumped through the right ventricle into the lungs, where carbon dioxide waste is removed and it is oxygenated, and then flows into the left atrium, the collecting chamber. Some of the oxygenated blood is used by the heart itself; the rest is pumped through the left ventricle into the circulatory system that serves the rest of the body. Deoxygenated blood (blood no longer containing oxygen and containing carbon dioxide) returns from the *vascular* (blood vessel) system to the right atrium, which feeds the right ventricle, and the cycle begins all over again. The circulatory system itself is composed of a complex network of pliable tubes through which blood flows, carrying oxygen and other nutrients to all organs and tissues of the body. These flexible blood vessels include *arteries* (which deliver fresh blood) and *veins* (which return deoxygenated and waste-filled products of metabolism to the heart). Small arteries are called *arterioles,* small veins are known as *venules.* The smallest blood vessels, which deliver blood to areas such as fingers and lung tissue, are called *capillaries.* In addition to delivering nutrients, blood circulation also helps in the disposal of toxins and other waste from the body's cells by filtering them through the kidneys and the lungs.

Because the cardiovascular system is literally the lifeline of the human body, any failure in its ability to perform places the brain, the kidneys, the heart itself, and potentially every organ and piece of tissue in the body at serious risk. In fact, it is safe to say that anything that threatens to keep your heart and circulatory system from its normal fueling process is a threat to your life. The heart, while being the most crucial of all our organs, is also, perhaps, the most resilient. As disturbing as the numbers are on heart disease and coronary death in America, I am amazed—as are many of my colleagues—that the numbers aren't higher, given the abuse that the average lifestyle inflicts on this never-resting muscle. Respect your heart as the strongest, most stoic part of your body, but listen to it and respond when it cries for help with a chest pain.

Cardiovascular disease is most often the outcome of one of —or any combination of—four things:

1. An impediment to the flow of blood through the heart itself.
2. An impediment to the flow of oxygenated blood from the lungs to the heart.
3. An impediment to the flow of blood somewhere else in the body.
4. A malfunctioning of the electrical system that triggers the pumping action—the heart's own natural pacemaker gone awry.

(Congenital heart defects, since these are dealt with during infancy and childhood, are not likely to be the cause of an adult chest pain.)

There are a number of heart maladies that can cause chest pain, from angina to valve disease to syphilitic heart disease to myocardial infarction. All are serious. All are potentially life-threatening; yet, all may be treatable, if dealt with in time. You cannot diagnose any of them yourself. My best advice to anyone having chest pain is to take action as if it were a coronary while hoping and praying that it is a minor valve disorder or one of the less serious noncardiac chest pains like reflux esophagitis.

Angina

What is angina and why does it cause chest pain?

Angina, medically known as *angina pectoris,* is an illness in which the heart, in trying to meet the oxygen demands of the body, becomes unable to meet its own oxygen demands. The pain itself is probably a function of the cellular deprivation of oxygen in the heart and the collection of metabolic byproducts (the exhaust of the heart's "fuel burning") that are not removed as fast as they should be. The pain is also a warning. Angina is a serious illness and can be the warning sign of an impending heart attack. It is estimated that nearly two and a half million Americans currently suffer from this oxygen insufficiency in the heart, including about 300,000 new cases per year, and almost all could probably have been prevented.

What exactly are the oxygen demands of the body?

Oxygen is the gasoline that fuels the cellular engines in your body. All enzymatic and life-functional processes that stoke your metabolic fire require oxygen. It is the fuel your body needs most urgently.

The oxygen demands of the body change, depending on your emotional and physical situation. When sleeping or relaxing, the body needs much less oxygen than when running, climbing stairs, worrying, or raging.

What causes the heart to be unable to meet this demand?

There are two major culprits. Blood that has, for unknown reasons, become too thick (or viscous) can hinder circulation and decrease oxygen supply to the heart. This is a relatively recent discovery. The other major culprit of angina is infamous. Arteriosclerotic blood vessels obstruct the flow of oxygenated blood. The heart pumps harder and harder to try and meet the oxygen demands of the body and, in doing so, increases its own oxygen need. If your blood vessels are arteriosclerotic, they cannot meet this increased demand.

What are arteriosclerotic blood vessels?

Arteriosclerosis, a medical term familiar to most Americans, means hardening of the arteries. The most common cause of arteriosclerosis is *atherosclerosis,* the degeneration of an artery caused by deposits of fat, cholesterol, fibrin (a blood-clotting material), cellular waste products, and calcium. Such vessels can completely close off.

How do these nasty deposits get there?

If the blood that passes through an artery is saturated with fats and cholesterol, some of these *lipid* (fat) molecules are left behind, like sludge or like grease at the bottom of a barbecue grill. This sludge, by the way, is not only the result of an excess saturated-fat diet but also of an elevated triglyceride level, which is aggravated by sugar molecules and other fat molecules in the blood and raised by coffee and alcohol. Being overweight also increases the amount of lipid molecules in the blood. Emotional stress may even play a significant role in cholesterol level and vascular disease, as I will discuss later in *The 50-Year Cholesterol and Hypertension Plan.* As this sludge begins to build up, it deposits calcium, fibrin, and cellular waste on the artery wall, which forms *plaque* (a plaster-like substance that hardens arteries).

There may be other contributory factors, such as immune system reactions to certain allergies and degeneration from wear and tear, but it is increasingly clear that for most people vascular disease is a disease of lifestyle. If atherosclerotic build-up occurs, as it does in the arteries of millions of Americans, eventually the areas of obstruction can severely restrict the flow of freshly oxygenated blood. Like lard poured down a kitchen sink, eventually it will obstruct the flow. If such plugging becomes complete, what you have on your hands —or I should say in your chest—is a full-blown heart attack. That's why the pain of angina can be a life-saving pain.

What about walking up stairs or running too fast? Doesn't that cause angina?

No. Increased activity raises the oxygen needs throughout the body, but it doesn't cause angina. If your cardiovascular system is healthy, you will never have angina pain—no matter how fast you run or how many stairs you walk up. Your muscles will not allow you to run fast enough to put an excess demand on your heart, if your heart is healthy. If your heart is sick enough, however, the simple act of lifting a suitcase can put an excess oxygen demand on the sick heart and can cause angina chest pain.

Exertion only brings on pain for an already-sick heart?

Yes. That is called stable angina, meaning there is pain with a certain degree of physical, emotional, or chemical change within the body. Often I hear patients talk about feeling chest pain while running to catch an airplane while carrying luggage. It is just as likely to be brought on by fear.

Fear increases the body's oxygen needs?

So do anger and other emotional conflict responses. It seems to have something to do with the fight-or-flight chemicals in the body. For example, you may consciously know that the traffic you are stuck in is not life-threatening, but the anger it is causing tells your body to be on guard, increasing adrenaline, increasing your heartbeat, and making your heart need more oxygen in order to pump at the increased rate. That is why panic disorder is so dangerous. It can *mimic* angina, and it can, in some cases, help *cause* angina. It can certainly bring on the pain of angina, and the only way to know what is going on is for a doctor to look and listen.

Sometimes physical exertion and emotional stress can combine for a really serious angina. The guy running to catch that plane might still be angry because he couldn't find a parking space, which is why he might miss the plane. Or, he might be fearful of what logistical horrors he will face if the plane takes off without him. Then he feels this chest pain and doesn't know whether to stop running or to try and ignore it, and the conflict within him makes the pain worsen. If he's smart, he'll stop running, drop his bags, and have someone in the airport get him medical attention.

Are there any other factors that bring on the pain of angina?

Inhaling cigarette smoke fills blood with carbon monoxide, which cannot coexist in the blood with oxygen. The carbon monoxide fixes itself to the hemoglobin-carrying molecule (that's the chemical in the blood that transports oxygen) and it won't let the oxygen on—like a rude passenger on a rush-hour subway train. The more carbon monoxide there is in the blood, the less oxygen. In some heavy smokers, levels of up to 20% carbon monoxide are found in the blood, which means oxygen is only 80% present. While the heart is pumping away, trying to meet the oxygen demands of the body, the blood it is pumping can be grossly lacking in oxygen. The heart has to keep working harder and harder to meet its oxygen demands. Cigarette smokers, garage workers, or anyone exposing themselves to heavy doses of carbon monoxide gases are all at risk. The long-term effects of breathing smog may produce this problem in some people.

Anemias can create a similar problem. Anemia is a deficiency of red blood cells, and red blood cells carry oxygen. Not enough red blood cells means not enough oxygen, which means the heart must work all that much harder to try and meet the body's oxygen demands.

What causes anemia?

Iron deficiency in the diet or an inability to absorb iron. Less common is a deficiency of vitamin B_{12} caused by an inherited lack of *intrinsic factor* (a chemical produced in the stomach cells necessary for the absorption of B_{12}) or other stomach problems. Vegetarians are also at risk for this kind of anemia because their diets are low in B_{12}. Pregnancy and excessive bleeding from ulcers and other conditions—many of which we have already discussed—may also result in anemias. So, ironically, can aspirin, which bleeds the stomach. I say ironic because aspirin is being touted now as a tool for preventing coronaries, if taken once a day or every other day. Although aspirin's potential side effects are, in some cases, outweighed by its benefits, it is imprudent to recommend it on a mass scale.

Are there still other potential causes of angina?

Possibly the second-most-common cause of angina is irregularity in heart rhythm. The pumping action of the heart is thus unable to do its part in delivering needed oxygen throughout the body effectively.

What causes heart rhythm irregularity?

The cause is arteriosclerotic plaquing of the blood vessels within the heart itself that feed oxygenated blood to the *Purkinje fibers* (the "electric wires" of the heart that bring the signal to the muscle cells and orchestrate the coordination of the contractions) or plaquing of blood vessels that serve the *sinus node* (the heart's natural pacemaker). Both obstructions will interrupt the heart's electrical system, as can defects or inadequacies within this "natural battery" within the heart. This "short circuiting" of the current that initiates the pumping action of the heart can give rise to irregular rhythms.

Irregular rhythm—isn't that a cardiac illness in and of itself?

Yes. And there are a number of other causes of arrhythmias that we will discuss in greater detail separately. All of them can bring on the pain of angina in anyone with atherosclerosis.

Have we left out any other potential causes of angina?

There are a number of other heart illnesses that can cause chest pain in and of themselves but that can also prevent the heart from meeting its oxygen demands and thus cause angina chest pain. These conditions include valve disorders, viral infections of the heart, cardiomyopathy, structural defects of the heart, and ventricular hypertrophy.

Pulmonary hypertension, which is a noncardiac condition capable of causing chest pain, can also cause angina by keeping the lungs from delivering the necessary oxygen to the heart. Any respiratory problem that denies the heart its needed oxygen (a common one is emphysema) can bring on the chest pain of angina.

Hyperthyroidism is another potential noncardiac cause of chest pain. An overactive thyroid gland, which produces too much thyroid hormone and speeds up the heart rate and increases its need for oxygen, can also cause angina pain in people with vascular disease. A disease called pheochromocytoma, which causes an excess of adrenaline in the body, can also make the heart go faster and blood pressure rise to exceptionally dangerous levels.

Any drug that increases heart rate, including caffeine, cocaine, and amphetamines, can also bring on angina chest pain.

Why are people with angina advised to move to a warmer climate?

Cold weather or even just a cold wind or draft brings on angina chest pain in people with vascular disease.

Why is that?

The same reason cold weather makes musical instruments play sharp. Heat expands matter by speeding up the kinetic energy of subatomic particles and cold shrinks matter by slowing down the kinetic energy of subatomic particles. Cold can shrink, therefore, the diameter of blood vessels. Normal, unplaqued vessels can adjust with minimal impact, but arteriosclerotic vessels can be restricted to the point of producing angina chest pain, when tightened by cold.

Any other exacerbating factors?

A high fever—especially a persistent one—can increase your circulatory oxygenation needs enough to bring on the pain of angina in an unhealthy heart muscle. So can overeating.

Overeating?

Digestion requires blood flow and oxygen delivery. Too much demand on stomach digestion at any one time means increased demand on the heart to pump blood. Overeating, as well as eating too fast or just eating too much fat at once, puts excess demand on stomach digestion. But don't replace excess food consumption with excess alcohol consumption.

Alcohol can also bring on angina?
In people with vascular disease, yes. Alcohol can stimulate fight-or-flight responses, raise adrenaline, cause irregular rhythms, or raise blood pressure. All of these effects can increase the heart's oxygen demands. Many over-the-counter medicines may also have this effect, especially diet pills. In addition to all of this, there are, as always, a number of idiopathic (or unknown) potential causes of angina.

You referred to stable angina. Is there an unstable angina?
Unfortunately, yes. Here's the difference. If the chest pain of angina subsides when the stimulus that initiated the increased oxygen demand ceases, this is stable angina. In other words, if you stop climbing the stairs or carrying the packages and stand still or rest or relax from the stressful emotions or quit smoking or treat the anemia or other root illness or get in out of the cold, the pain should be relieved. In stable angina, the pain gets worse depending on the severity of its stimulus, and it usually responds to nitroglycerin treatment or any other treatment that dilates blood vessels.

Unstable angina refers to an angina that causes greater and greater pain from less and less oxygen demand over time. For example, someone who used to feel chest pain carrying two bags of groceries and walking home might now feel a much worse pain just from lifting one bag of groceries and taking one step. The most serious extreme of this is called "angina at rest" and refers to an angina pain that just happens without an increase in oxygen demand. It usually indicates that arteries are at least 70% obstructed. Unstable angina of any degree is a medical emergency that requires immediate hospitalization. It can be the beginning of an acute heart attack.

How does the chest pain of angina feel?

It is almost always substernal—just under the breastbone—and almost always is defined in certain very specific terms. Angina patients, when able to pinpoint and describe their pain, often describe a tightness in the chest or a crushing feeling in the chest, as if someone were walking on it or as if a thousand pounds of lead were sitting on it. Sometimes it is compared to a heavy blow, which in some cases eases up, in some cases does not. I have also had patients describe a sharp knifing pain and other kinds of pain that turned out to be angina. I cannot really say whether they were inaccurately describing what they were feeling or not. It is, after all, a stressful and often dizzying situation.

Sometimes the pain isn't even in the chest. Angina pain can afflict the wrists, the shoulders, the nose, the chin, and the jaw. It is commonly mistaken for a toothache. I have known dentists who, unable to find a dental explanation for a patient's toothache, have sent the patient to a cardiologist and possibly saved the patient's life. If you ever get a chin pain from climbing stairs or a toothache from playing tennis or if your wrists hurt when you get angry or your shoulders or jaw ache when something scares you, see a doctor immediately.

Is there any known reason why angina can cause pain in these other places?

Often there is confusion of multiple pain nerve tracts that fail to define the main locus of pain. Pain seems more easily reported by the brain when it occurs on our skin than within our bodies.

What is the treatment of angina?

First we have to make the diagnosis. I always hope that the patient describes the pain accurately so that we can begin to suspect angina and can look for it. If not, I would always get an *electrocardiogram* (EKG), which measures the rhythm of the heart, the normal oxygenation of the heart, problems in oxygenating the heart, and any dead tissue from coronary or *myocardial infarction* (the damaging or death of an area of the heart muscle resulting from a reduced blood supply to that area). If the angina is stable, the problem may not show up on the initial EKG. We may need to put the patient on a treadmill and increase the body's oxygen demands in order to expose any stable angina.

When I see a man (for some reason, it's always a man) on a TV medical news show walking and walking and getting nowhere with wires coming out of his chest . . . ?

Exactly. That's an electrocardiogram on a treadmill. Now, if further diagnosis is needed, a thalium scan test is administered while the patient is on a treadmill, in which a radioactive chemical called thalium-201 is injected into the bloodstream at the peak of physical exertion. Through X-ray technology, we can follow the flow of this liquid and see how the blood is passing through the system and find any dead tissue or complete obstruction.

And this stuff is radioactive?

Yes, but we use a very tiny amount for the test. The cancer risk is minimal—less than your average set of dental X rays—and the potential health benefit of a proper cardiac diagnosis far exceeds this risk.

If angina is diagnosed, what then?

The first and most immediate line of defense is usually nitroglycerin, referred to by many doctors as TNT because it is a nonexplosive form of the famous explosive chemical.

Nitroglycerin is a vasodilator, which means it dilates (or expands) blood vessels, whether they are contracted from cold or clogged from plaque. If the angina is the stable type, nitroglycerin almost always relieves the chest pain. Unstable angina will sometimes respond to TNT. Angina at rest will not.

Is this a pill you take?

For years nitroglycerin was administered under the tongue. Recent advances have come up with a nitroglycerin patch for the skin over the troubled blood vessels and nitroglycerin paste that is applied to rice paper with measurement diagrams and placed on the skin. The nitroglycerin is absorbed through the skin into the blood vessels and dilates them. These patches and paste applications last up to 24 hours, then must be replaced. There is also another drug called isosorbide, which performs a similar function. Like nitroglycerin, it is usually taken under the tongue.

It is important to remember, however, that these drugs represent stopgap measures. They can ease pain and, for a time, prevent the blockage that can lead to a heart attack. But they are not a long-term solution. The only long-term solution to atherosclerosis is a change in lifestyle. The same recommendations I make to anyone wanting to *avoid* heart disease must be followed by anyone wishing to *recover* from heart disease, beginning with lowering the level of blood cholesterol to 160. These dilating drugs are likely to stop being effective in overcoming the arterial obstruction. Thus stable or unstable angina can lead to a heart attack or, at the very least, to bypass surgery.

Bypass surgery? Isn't that what happens after the heart attack?

Not necessarily. Sometimes your doctor can find vascular disease that has progressed so far that a heart attack is imminent, though you luckily have not had it yet. He or she can open you up and reroute the circulation within the heart, much the way a plumber would reroute water around an obstructed pipe. And yet, bypass surgery, although life-saving, is merely a temporary treatment. Blood vessel disease, if not dealt with through diet, exercise, and other lifestyle changes, can still kill you.

Bypass surgery and vasodilators are a temporary solution?

Yes, and as for the nitrate-dilating drugs, such as nitroglycerin, the less often they need to be used *the better,* because there may be a long-term cancer risk and short-term headache problems.

Why is that?

Chemically, nitrate medicines are the same as the nitrates commonly used in foods (to keep lettuce crisp at the salad bar and to keep the color of processed meats vivid). These nitrates combine with protein in the stomach to form carcinogenic nitrosamines. Of course, the benefits of these drugs in saving the lives of heart patients are often worth this long-term risk. In order to diminish the risk for my patients, I always prescribe a 250-milligram tablet of vitamin C along with any dosage of nitroglycerin, isosorbide, or any other nitrate heart medicine because vitamin C seems to deactivate nitrosamine.

As for headaches, any substance that dilates blood vessels in the cardiac area can also dilate blood vessels in the head, causing agonizing headaches in some people.

Are there any nonnitrate medicines available?

Some medicines that have recently come into wide use for angina include beta blockers, which can prevent the sudden burst of adrenaline triggered by fear, anger, anxiety, and other highly charged emotions. Since adrenaline and its products speed up the heart and can cause angina in people with heart disease, blocking this adrenal dumping can be part of the temporary treatment of angina. Some well-known beta blockers are Inderal, Lopressor, Tenormin, and Corgard.

Another very popular new group of medicines are the calcium channel blockers, which have become about as commonly used in the treatment of heart disease as aspirin. Calcium channel blockers work in two ways. They are excellent dilators of blood vessels and can keep the oxygen flowing and help stabilize heart rhythms. The most commonly used ones are diltiazem, verapamil, and nifedipine.

And they block calcium?

Not dietary calcium. In other words, they do not hinder the absorption of calcium, and so they don't increase the risk of osteoporosis and other bone disease. They do prevent calcium ion exchange in the cells of blood vessels. Calcium ion exchange is what chemically causes vessels to go into spasms and thus reduce in diameter. In effect, blocking this ion exchange dilates the blood vessels.

Are any other medications used?

Two other commonly used heart medicines are hydrolazine and captopril. Hydrolazine brings blood pressure down and can relieve angina pain. Captopril helps prevent blood vessel contractions, helping to prevent heart attacks and even giving strength to the heart.

Of course, these medicines are invaluable and can literally save lives, but, as with any drugs, there are known and unknown side effects. Let your doctor use them for as long as it is necessary but do your part to overcome heart disease with lifestyle changes and limit your need for all these medicines.

What if none of these work?

If a major obstruction can be found, we will often try what is called an *angioplasty balloon*. Because it is more like a plumbing snake, I like to call it a cardiac roto-rooter. It's a sponge-like surgical device on the end of a catheter that is passed through the blood vessels and can often push through the sludge and clear it out. Of course, the patient must decide if he or she wants to change his or her lifestyle so that other such obstructions don't have to be plowed away continually. The balloon is a wonderful life-saving technology, but, as with anything in medicine, it carries no guarantee, and there is a risk.

What's the risk?

There is a relatively small—but not insignificant—risk that this medical intervention can actually *cause* a coronary thrombosis or heart attack.

And if the balloon doesn't work?

If an angina patient has not responded to nitroglycerin or other medicines and has not responded to a change in lifestyle and is unable to be treated with a balloon, bypass surgery is usually the next step. For that matter, anyone under 40 with angina or anyone who has had a heart attack and whose angina pain is not relieved through any of the available medicines must consider this step as well.

It is important to know that when your doctor prescribes an angiogram, which involves the passage of dye through the blood vessels, it is very likely that a surgery team and a table are waiting for you. An angiogram not only determines the need for the operation but also determines what area the surgery needs to be performed on—and it's not a decision that can wait. So, if you have angina and it's not responding to medications or a balloon, or if your doctor asks you whether you're following a low-cholesterol diet, walking, managing your stress, and quitting smoking and you say yes but it's not quite the truth, or even if you just haven't been properly taking the prescribed medicines, it may be time for some honesty with your doctor and with yourself.

Cardiac bypass surgery has a significantly high rate of success. In fact a recent study found the short-term death rate was lower among those who've had bypass surgery than those treated with medication only, though the short-term death rates for both are, happily, quite small. However, surgery is always a risk and recovery is never easy. Moreover, if a change in lifestyle does not *follow* this kind of surgery, then you are in *big* trouble. The new heart circulatory routes will plug up even faster than the old ones if cholesterol is not controlled, and within two to five years you could need another bypass. So, always be honest with yourself and with your doctor to help him or her make the right therapeutic decision for your illness.

With surgery and/or medicines and with a change in lifestyle, you can treat your angina before it closes up into a heart attack. A pain in your chest may be trying to tell you to do just that. You can also treat your angina before it gets any worse. If you don't have angina you can, through the preventive measures I discuss later, keep from ever suffering from this life-threatening and life-hindering disease.

Heart Irregularity

What are heart irregularities?

Arrhythmia, as it is medically referred to, is simply any abnormal rhythm of the heart. This is not to say that each person's *normal* rhythm is the same or that heart rhythms don't normally change.

What is a normal range?

At rest, it is between 70 and about 84 beats per minute (bpm). Exercise or anxiety—or other good and bad stresses —can raise the heart rate to as much as 80% of its healthy maximum. Although the at-rest heart rate does not normally change, the maximum changes with age. At 35 years old, it is about 148 bpm. At 65, it is about 124 bpm. This speeding up and slowing down of the heart's contractions, even when it does go from its healthy slow to 80% of its healthy maximum, is normally done in a steady, coordinated fashion, like a drummer changing rhythms with a clean transition so as not to upset the other musicians.

What constitutes an irregularity?

Anything that violates one or more of those norms, slower than normal at rest, faster than the healthy maximum, or inconsistent and uncoordinated.

There are a number of specific arrhythmias. They are defined by location and type. Locations are atrial (the top part of the heart) and ventricular (the bottom part of the heart). Types are *tachycardia* (irregularly rapid heartbeats of between 130 and 150 bpm); *fibrillation* (dangerously uncoordinated contractions of the heart muscle causing heartbeats so irregular that they are difficult to measure), the most common arrythmia; *flutter* (irregular beats that go so fast, as much as 300 bpm, that the heart may not be able to contract fully; and *bradycardia* (a dangerously slow heart rhythm of less than 60 bpm). In bradycardia, the rhythm can drop as low as 30 bpm, a medical emergency, or slower, potentially causing a person to faint and ultimately go into *cardiac arrest* (the heart stops beating).

What causes all these problems?

Probably the most common causes are problems in the body's electrical system.

Is that the same sinus node and Purkinje fibers that we discussed before?

That's right. And the most common problem in this electrical system is, as we discussed, arteriosclerosis of the vessels serving the Purkinje fibers. If not dealt with this problem can not only cause angina pectoris but also any number of heart irregularities and associated chest pain. In fact, if the arteriosclerosis is left untreated for a period of time, it can lead to sick sinus syndrome, in which the sinus node becomes irreversibly diseased and useless as a regulator of heart rhythm.

Can anything be done about it?

Fortunately, an artificial pacemaker can now be implanted and take the place of the sick sinus node. This artificial pacemaker runs on a battery that can last between five and eight years. The operation has a relatively low risk, and most people with pacemakers can resume normal active lives—if they change their lifestyle to try and prevent further cardiac complications. The pacemaker must be monitored regularly to make sure it's regulating heart rhythms accurately, and even though the newer pacemakers have a high degree of reliability and have saved and extended the lives of thousands of people, no machine is quite as reliable as a healthy heart.

What other conditions cause these heart electrical problems?

Like many other kinds of electrical generators, the heart's signal-producing mechanism uses specific ions (electrically charged atoms) derived from certain minerals to produce electricity. In particular, the heart needs a proper balance of potassium, sodium, calcium, and magnesium. That's why joggers on very low-calorie diets sometimes collapse from heart failure. By jogging they sweat out what little potassium and salt they have. Any imbalance in these minerals—caused by severe inadequacy or excess—can compromise the pumping action of the heart. Like a car battery without enough water or acid, it just won't work properly.

What do I do to make sure I don't have such an imbalance?

First, let me tell you what not to do. Don't use this as a reason to consume excess amounts of salt. Excess salt, as I will discuss later, can increase the risk of high blood pressure.

As for what to do, fortunately these much-needed minerals can be found in a wide assortment of fruits and vegetables. In addition, if you follow my suggested plan for vitamin and mineral insurance in the preventive section, you can greatly reduce the risk of imbalance. But don't ingest megadoses of vitamins and minerals—especially vitamin D, which can deplete potassium, calcium, and magnesium.

Any other causes of irregular heart rhythms?

Anxiety and other emotional conditions can cause spontaneous heartbeat irregularities, as can caffeine. Often a patient will complain of all the symptoms of irregular heart rhythms, but I cannot find any damage to the heart's electrical system. The first question I will ask is, "Are you feeling an unusual amount of anxiety lately?" The next question: "How many cups of coffee or cola do you drink each day?" Caffeine-induced irregularities are usually reversible once you cut down or quit caffeine consumption. Cocaine, alcohol, and many other drugs, however, can cause permanent irregularities, as well as serious heart muscle damage.

Other causes of arrhythmias include pericarditis and *febrile illnesses* (any illness producing temperature elevation) such as pneumonia.

What kind of chest pain do these heart irregularities cause?

Usually it is an angina-like pain with shortness of breath, light-headedness, a feeling of faintness, perspiration, and general weakness.

What is the treatment?

If the irregularity is at a dangerous level, emergency measures must often be employed. Electric shock can sometimes regulate a newly formed fibrillation. This is known as cardioversion. Medicines such as digitalis and propanalol may also be used to regulate heart rhythms.

Long-term treatment can be planned once we have isolated the root cause. Then, we can treat arrhythmia by removing this cause or dealing with it—that is, treat the pneumonia, relax, stop drinking ten cups of coffee and five cans of cola each day, and so on.

In addition to lifestyle changes, medicines such as digitalis, quinidine, beta blockers, calcium channel blockers, and procaine may sometimes be necessary to help regulate irregular heart rhythms on an ongoing basis.

If these medicines are unable to regulate heart rhythms and lifestyle changes are ineffective—or come too little and too late—then a pacemaker is the next consideration.

Pericarditis

What is pericarditis?

It's an inflammation of the pericardium. The pericardium is the plastic wrap–like sac which encloses the heart. It is composed of two layers, an outer fibrous pericardium and a thin inner serous pericardium. The pericardium protects the heart, and lubrication between the two layers provides for smooth contractions. But sometimes the pericardium can become injured, inflamed, infected, or even tumorous —much the same way that the pleura can.

What kind of injuries can happen to the pericardium?

Common injuries include any piercing of the chest, from a car accident or a knife wound. The sharp edge of a fractured rib can also injure the pericardium.

How does the pericardium become inflamed?

It can be inflamed as part of a *systemic illness* (an illness affecting different parts of the body at the same time), such as rheumatoid arthritis, lupus, or even uremia.

Sometimes pericardial inflammation can be a side effect of a drug. Procaine (a common heart medicine), hydrolazine (an antihypertension medicine), and Dilantin (an antiseizure medicine) are examples of drugs with such potential side effects. Pericarditis can even be a symptom of a coronary, and in some cases it is the pericardial inflammation that gets the patient to the hospital where the *myocardial infarction* (heart attack) can be treated.

Usually, however, we are not really sure what causes pericardial inflammation.

What causes pericardial infection?

Viruses and bacteria are often the culprits, as well as other idiopathic causes.

Are pericardial tumors of any particular nature?

Lymphomas (tumors of the lymphatic system), *sarcomas* (tumors of the muscular system), or *metastasized tumors* (tumors spread throughout the body) are most common.

What kind of chest pain does pericarditis cause?

Pericarditis usually causes a steady, mid-chest pain under the sternum. Lying down, especially on the left side, will often make it worse. Sitting up usually relieves the pain to some degree. Sometimes the pain can radiate to the shoulders or up to the neck. I have heard this pain described as sharp, dull, mild, and very serious. It all depends on the person, the type of irritation, and the severity; regretfully, a tumor often causes no pain and can therefore go unnoticed. Pericarditis pain sometimes gets worse with breathing, coughing, and sneezing. Often any movement will make it worse. This is one way a doctor can rule out a heart attack in cases of pericarditis, because heart attack pain neither worsens nor lessens with movement. The chills and fever that often accompany pericarditis are not often associated with a heart attack either.

If there are no chills or fever, how does a doctor make the right diagnosis?

Sometimes listening with a stethoscope, we can hear friction, like leaves rubbing against each other in the wind, which may be the two layers of the pericardium rubbing against each other, telling us there is pericarditis. An *echocardiogram* (a sound-wave reading of the heart) can also be helpful along with an electrocardiogram, X ray, and an angiogram through the aorta into the heart. If *tamponade* (collection of blood or other non-pericardial fluid in the pericardial sac that constricts the heart) is suspected, we can usually make a diagnosis by measuring the *wedge pressure* (the blood pressure within the heart itself).

It is very important that you get this condition diagnosed immediately. Pericarditis is a serious condition. Not just because of the possibility of cancer. Pericarditis can cause tissue to become scarred or swollen, or the two pericardial layers can become stuck together, which can compress the heart and/or make contraction impossible. But none of this has to happen if it's diagnosed and treated quickly.

What's the treatment for pericarditis?

It's an intensive care situation, and so you must waste no time in getting medical attention. If we can identify the cause—arthritis, drug reaction, tumors, infection, or underlying heart condition—we will treat it while relieving pain with medication and anxiety with a little reassurance. Sometimes, if there is hemorrhaging, the sac will fill with blood and cause sac enlargement. In that case, we might need to surgically drain all this excess fluid with a procedure called pericardicentesis. If not, nonsteroidal antiinflammatory drugs or cortisone are often used. Bed rest is a must, with diuretics and oxygen administered if necessary. Antibiotics and time can usually heal the inflammation. A low-salt diet is often prescribed to relieve blood pressure and blood volume, which relieves the workload of the heart.

Myocarditis

What is myocarditis?

An inflammation of the muscle cells that compose the heart and that contract to perform the pumping action. It is a potentially serious, though most often not life-threatening, condition.

What causes it?

Myocarditis can be caused by a viral or bacterial infection, by a systemic illness such as rheumatoid arthritis, or by other collagen disease such as lupus. Myocarditis can also be a complication of such diseases as second- and third-stage syphilis. It is even possible that a pericardial or pleural infection, if not treated, can spread to the heart and cause this inflammation.

What kinds of viruses cause myocarditis?

Any virus can. No one is really sure why a virus might end up infecting the heart (or any other part of the body, for that matter). It just happens. Some common viruses associated with this illness are the herpes virus group, including the Epstein-Barr virus, the cytomegalovirus, and Coxsackie virus. Polio, a virus that has been made virtually extinct in the United States, is (or was) notorious for liking to settle into the cardiac muscle.

How commonly will a common flu virus infection cause myocarditis?

No one, as far as I know, has ever calculated that. But I would suspect it is relatively rare, rare enough not to cause panic the next time you think you have the flu, though you still need to take good care of yourself to ensure recovery from the flu.

Does anyone know how or why systemic illness and syphilis cause inflammation of the heart?

Not really. In the case of systemic illnesses, it may be a confusion within the immune system of antibody chemicals. Syphilis is just a nasty disease that can inflict a whole set of horrors on its victims.

What kind of chest pain does myocarditis cause?

Nothing specific. In fact, myocarditis is usually a diagnosis made after most other cardiac illnesses have been ruled out. As with many other cardiac illnesses, myocarditis can cause shortness of breath and increased heart rate along with chest pain. Sometimes the patient also suffers from fever and fatigue, which tend to be more specifically characteristic of myocarditis. The symptoms do not seem to vary with regard to cause, although the intensity of inflammation and muscle deterioration is far greater from syphilitic myocarditis. Myocarditis resulting from second-stage syphilis can cause sudden death.

What's the treatment?

We treat the cause. If the cause is bacterial, we will use antibiotics. Virally caused myocarditis is treated with bed rest, fluids, and support. Sometimes we administer cortisone and antiinflammatory medicines. If the cause is a systemic illness, diagnosis becomes all the more critical; we use antiinflammatory agents or antiimmune agents. For second-stage syphilis, penicillin or a drug called doxycycline is often used. Of course, the best way to treat syphilis is long before it reaches the second stage. Treat it now! Third-stage syphilis can cause still other serious heart illnesses.

Syphilitic Heart Disease

I've heard you can go blind and crazy from syphilis. Are you telling me that there can also be heart disease?

Second- and third-stage syphilis can cause very serious heart disease.

What do you mean "second- and third-stage" syphilis?

Syphilis, like many other venereal diseases, goes into latency after its initial onset, then can return in a much more severe form. That's second stage. On the average, it happens nine months to one year after the onset of the syphilis. Most people survive this second stage, which then goes into latency only to return 20 or 25 years later as a potentially fatal disease, including heart disease.

What kind of heart disease?

Third-stage syphilis can cause *aortitis* (an inflammation of the inside lining of the aorta) and aortic aneurism. Second- or third-stage syphilis can cause obliterative endarteritis of the vasa vasorum (small nutrient arteries and veins), which is an inflammation of one of the layers of the aorta and the capillaries serving that area. Endarteritis can, in turn, bring on disease of the valve between the aorta and the heart. If there is valve involvement, then syphilitic heart disease can even bring on congestive heart failure.

With these aortic and valve disorders, what kind of chest pain is there?

Nothing specific. In fact diagnosis is often extremely difficult because many doctors won't think about syphilis as the underlying cause. It may ultimately be up to the patient to consider that he or she might have once contracted syphilis and never dealt with it.

How would I know if I contracted it?

It takes a pretty good memory. Remember, third-stage syphilis happens about twenty-five years after you first contract this venereal disease. And, unlike most other venereal diseases, the initial symptoms are usually not serious. A hard *chancre* (ulceration) will appear on the genitalia, mouth, or virtually any other part of the body. It is painless, however, and seems superficial, even though it is not. Sometimes the ulcer is so small it can be dismissed as a pimple. Sometimes the only symptom is a swollen lymph node, which is hardly the kind of thing that makes people assume they have contracted a venereal disease. Second-stage syphilis, which occurs in at least one out of every three cases, is the body's attempt to get rid of the illness. This happens anywhere from one to nine months after the first stage of the disease. Symptoms can range from headaches, to bone and joint pain, baldness, conjunctivitis, hepatitis, kidney disorders, meningitis, and myocarditis—none of which immediately bring venereal disease to mind—or it can be as minimal as a painless rash. After about two years, virtually all second-stage symptoms disappear. The disease then remains in latency for up to twenty or twenty-five years, when it can cause problems, including potentially fatal heart disease.

SYPHILITIC HEART DISEASE

Syphilis is an illness that has been all but forgotten, but in the last few years we are seeing more cases in the United States than we have in more than a decade.

How are the heart diseases caused by second- and third-stage syphilis treated?

Surgically and, if treated soon enough, with moderate success. Unfortunately, the statistics for survival and longevity with regard to third-stage syphilis complications have been somewhat bleak, which is all the more reason to deal with the disease before it gets this far. These heart maladies, when caused by syphilis, are far more intense. Furthermore, if the heart ailment is dealt with surgically but the syphilis is still not diagnosed and treated, you are left vulnerable to recurring illness and possible sudden death.

What can I do to make sure that I never catch the disease in the first place?

At the risk of repeating a cliché, safe sex, which at the moment means monogamy and/or use of condoms.

If I think I might have contracted syphilis some years ago, is there any way I can find out and have it treated before I get heart disease?

Yes, by all means, if you have any suspicion, your doctor can do blood tests that might possibly show the presence of a latent syphilis, which can be dealt with well before it reaches the third stage.

Left Ventricular Hypertrophy

What is left ventricular hypertrophy?

It is an illness in which the left ventricle, the one pumping blood out of the heart and into the body's circulatory system, enlarges. This abnormal enlargement, if allowed to proceed unchecked, can make the heart larger than its contractile efficiency can support. In other words, it gets bigger but it doesn't get stronger. Thus the enlarged heart cannot keep up with the body's demand for oxygen or supply its own oxygen needs, which can cause congestive heart failure, often with associated chest pain. It can be a very serious condition and can lead to irregular rhythms and heart attack.

What causes this abnormal enlargement?

Probably the most common cause is hypertension (high blood pressure), often caused by an excess of fluid in the circulatory system though it can also occur when blood vessels contract or spasm (because of intense fear or anger or other reason) on an otherwise normal level of circulatory fluid. Either way, hypertension causes increased pressure on the heart's pumping action.

This increased pressure causes heart muscle tension —the way pumping iron tenses muscles in the arms or legs or back or wherever, depending on what kind of weight-lifting exercises you are doing. Just as your biceps, triceps, and deltoids enlarge from this steady increase of tension, so does the left ventricle become larger from the increased tension of high blood pressure.

I've heard that aerobic exercise also enlarges the heart. Isn't this dangerous?

No. When you exercise, you strengthen the heart muscle and pumping action and, yes, you can also enlarge it. The difference is that enlargement from exercise is in balance with the rest of your physiology, supported by increased cardiopulmonary ability to deliver sufficient oxygen to keep up with the increased demand. When enlargement is from hypertension, this increased oxygen delivery does not occur.

What kind of chest pain does left ventricular hypertrophy cause?

Unfortunately, it is usually painless—and therefore difficult to diagnose. When it is painful, it is most often identical to the pain of angina, given that both are conditions in which the heart cannot meet its own oxygen demands.

What is the treatment for left ventricular hypertrophy?

Treatment is twofold:
1. Treat the hypertension. This is done either by reducing circulatory fluid, with a low-sodium diet and diuretics if necessary, or by controlling blood-vessel spasms with dilating medicines such as nitroglycerin and calcium channel blockers.
2. Strengthen the heart muscles with safely regulated amounts of cardiovascular exercise and medicines such as digitalis or captopril.

Is it possible to diagnose and treat left ventricular hypertrophy before it causes congestive heart failure?

Absolutely. We need to discover whether there is associated valve disease and, if so, treat it surgically. Otherwise, the treatment for left ventricular hypertrophy is the treatment of the high blood pressure that caused it. Once blood pressure is lowered, the heart will usually correct itself. In fact, it is possible to diagnose and treat high blood pressure before it even causes left ventricular hypertrophy!

How can I do that?

To begin with, by bringing the silent killer out of hiding. You can take your own blood pressure at home or at the very least, see your doctor regularly so that he or she can catch high blood pressure, which is anything in excess of 145/85, and get you on hypertension therapy.

What is hypertension therapy?

It's a lifestyle change. It involves changes in diet, in activity, and in stress reduction. It may be nothing more than losing weight and walking every day. In addition, medicines such as diuretics can be used to help reduce blood pressure.

Valve Disorders

What are heart valves and what can go wrong with them?

There are four different valves within the heart, each consisting of several membranous flaps. They keep the blood flowing in the right direction. They are the mitral valve, the aortic valve, the tricuspid valve, and the pulmonary valve. Two problems common to these valves are prolapse and stenosis or insufficiency.

What is valve prolapse?

The function of these valves is to open and close, which regulates the flow of blood into and out of the heart. *Prolapse* refers to a condition in which a valve falls back out of its normal position, diminishing the efficiency of the valve. The most common valve prolapse occurs in the mitral valve. In that case, a leaflet of the valve falls back toward the ventricle and can inhibit the heart's efficiency at pumping blood into the circulatory system.

Are there any known causes?

Rheumatic fever in children can cause any of the valve illnesses (though often the valve disorder is not discovered until adulthood), but the most common kind of valve prolapse we see today occurs in adults who have never had rheumatic fever. We don't know the cause; it is probably an inherited predisposition. What seems to happen is that one of the valve pods starts to prolapse (push backwards) slightly, causing mitral or other *valve regurgitation* (leakage backwards). This regurgitation, which in the case of mitral valve prolapse is leaking back into the left ventricle, is often small and can be asymptomatic (usually a sign that the illness is usually not problematic).

And if a valve prolapse is not asymptomatic, what kind of chest pain does it cause?

Vague pressure or a sensation of fullness in the chest are common chest pains associated with valve disorders. Other symptoms include shortness of breath, recurring dizziness, fatigue, and panic. Often patients notice that their heartbeat becomes more noticeable, though not necessarily painful. What they're describing is a heart palpitation.

How is it diagnosed?

Often we can hear a mitral valve or other valve prolapse; we listen for a systolic murmur (an abnormal sound caused by a change in the configuration of blood flow) from the mitral or other valve. If we hear it or if we suspect for any reason that there is mitral or other valve prolapse, we do an echocardiogram, a sound-wave reading of the heart on which we can usually see such a prolapse.

What's the treatment?

If there is a significant leak, then we will want to surgically repair or replace part or all of the mitral valve. Most mitral valve prolapses do not require surgical repair.

What are the dangers of regurgitation?

Again, in most cases there is no regurgitation. But valves that do leak large amounts of blood back into the heart can cause overexertion of the heart and subsequent enlargement of the heart or one of its ventricles, much the way hypertension causes left ventricular hypertrophy. Fatigue and dizziness are very common with excessive regurgitation, because more blood is often leaking back than moving forward into the body's circulatory system. I have heard it described as "feeling like I just got out of bed—all day long."

And if there is prolapse without regurgitation?

Often we choose not to do surgery, though the condition must be monitored in case a leak does begin and the patient needs to take certain precautions in order to avoid valvulitis.

What's valvulitis?

It's a microorganistic infection in the valve, usually caused by a virus or bacteria. This illness can happen whenever microbacteria deposit upon a valve that is damaged or prolapsed. That's why if you are diagnosed as having mitral or other valve prolapse without regurgitation, your doctor will always tell you to get a prescription of antibiotic (be sure to take it) whenever you go to the dentist—even just for a cleaning.

Why is that?

Because dental manipulation or cleaning can often cause microscopic incisions in well-capillaried gums, allowing unwanted entry of bacteria into the bloodstream, and these nasty little critters seem to prefer to settle on a prolapsed mitral or other valve, causing this illness. Left untreated, this is a potentially fatal illness, but it can be prevented by a doctor's prescription of oral antibiotic.

Are there any other precautions I would want to take to prevent this disease if I have mitral valve prolapse?

If you ever experience any significant abscess, laceration, or injury to any part of your body, it would be important to remind the treating physician that you have mitral valve prolapse, in case there is any risk of exposure to microbacteria.

You've helped me understand prolapse. Now, what is valvular stenosis?

It's the opposite of a prolapse. Whereas a prolapse prevents the valve from being able to close fully, stenosis is a build-up of fibrous tissue which prevents the valve from being able to open fully and can thus severely slow down or completely obstruct the flow of blood. The most common such obstruction is mitral valve stenosis, which blocks the flow of blood from the lungs into the heart.

What causes this fibrous tissue to build up?

No one is sure. In some cases it is the result of rheumatic fever. Other times we just don't know.

What kind of chest pain does valvular stenosis cause?

Nothing specific. Much depends on the degree of closure of the valve and the progression of the problem. Because the pain is often caused by a resulting pulmonary hypertension, the pain can often be described in those terms. Other symptoms include fatigue and shortness of breath, which can get so severe that sleeping or lying down becomes impossible.

Obviously, this is a very serious condition. Without treatment, you run the risk of heart failure.

How is stenosis treated?

With immediate medical attention to stabilize respiration and circulation. Ultimately, the valve must be surgically opened to its normal position.

Bacterial Endocarditis

Isn't bacterial endocarditis what you have to watch out for if you have mitral valve prolapse and go to the dentist?

Exactly, but the dentist's chair is not the only place bacterial endocarditis strikes, and the mitral and other valves aren't the only places where the infection can occur. Various bacteria that enter your body in any number of ways can settle in the inner lining of the heart known as the endocardium. It can be an aftereffect of surgery, during which some bacteria may sneak their way from your own body's surface or intestines into your blood system. Streptococcus, enterovirus, and gonorrheal bacteria (yes, gonorrhea, as in "the clap") are microorganisms often found infecting the heart's inner lining.

And this causes chest pain?

Yes, though usually it is a later symptom, taking a backseat to chills, fever, and other flu-like symptoms. Joint pains are also a common early symptom. I hope you're the kind of person who takes a flu seriously enough to see the doctor, in which case early diagnosis and treatment of bacterial endocarditis are possible using antibiotics, bed rest, fluids, and good nutrition.

Cardiomyopathy

What is cardiomyopathy?

It is a very general term encompassing any illness specific to a heart muscle. Heart muscle illness can diminish the capacity of the heart's pumping action, cause rhythm irregularities, and cause heart failure.

Are there any known causes?

Yes, and many unknown causes. About half of all cardiomyopathies are the result of a viral infection. Less common causes include excess alcohol consumption, probably because alcohol's first metabolic breakdown product (the first chemical alcohol converts to during digestion) is acetaldehyde, a known toxin to muscle cells; exposure to lead and other poisons; the side effects of a host of toxic substances and drugs; exposure to cobalt, a metal sometimes added to beer as a foam stabilizer; thiamine deficiency, common in teenagers who eat too many processed foods and don't exercise sufficiently; deficiency in the amino acid L-carnitine; heavy exercise without proper nutrition; and excess adrenaline released within the body.

What kind of chest pain does cardiomyopathy cause?

Nothing specific. Any kind of chest pain could potentially turn out to be cardiomyopathy, even a very intense and debilitating chest pain.

How are cardiomyopathies treated?

According to the cause. If the cause is viral, we treat the virus and the general body system. In the event of toxic exposure, which includes alcohol and beer containing cobalt, we administer appropriate antidotes along with the slow intravenous infusion of fluids and nutrients where indicated and appropriate treatment to rid the body of the particular toxin or toxins. If a cardiomyopathy is the side effect of a drug, the drug is replaced with a different drug to be monitored for potentially similar side effects. If the cause is nutritional, such as a B vitamin, mineral, or protein deficiency, we look at diet modifications or the possibility of metabolic absorption problems, which may turn out to be a drug side effect. Interestingly, in many cases of cardiomyopathy where age seems to be a factor, when nutritional deficiencies are dealt with the problem usually stabilizes; sometimes it even goes away. In any case, while treating the cause, we always have to watch for possible arrhythmias. We also might use such medicines as cortisone and verapamil and many others in order to reduce inflammation and to make the heart muscle more efficient and stronger and to maintain blood pressure and healthy circulation.

Cardiac Tumors

Are cardiac tumors cancer of the heart?

Yes. Benign and malignant tumors do grow on the heart. Fortunately, heart cancers are rare. They are more common in children than in adults, which may or may not be comforting to you.

And they cause chest pain?

Sometimes. Nothing specific. And the chest pain may help in early detection. There are usually no other symptoms.

What is the treatment?

The tumor must be removed. Even if it is benign and it is allowed to grow on the heart muscle, it can severely interfere with circulation. The smaller it is when your doctor finds it, the greater your chances of survival.

Heart Attack

What exactly is a heart attack?

We've already talked about the heart's not getting enough oxygen to meet its own demands. When the heart, or a part of the heart, is completely cut off from the flow of oxygenated blood by a clot, any heart muscle beyond the point of the clot can die. This death of heart muscle is known as a heart attack (also known as a coronary thrombosis or a myocardial infarction).

And this is the result of arteriosclerosis?

Yes. The complete obstruction of a blood vessel within the heart can result from a blood clot forming or snagging in a heavily plaqued area. The blockage can also result from cholesterol or calcium plaque that completely obstructs the vessel; at such closures, a blood clot will always form.

Are there causes other than plaque and cholesterol? Don't people have heart attacks from severe emotional shock or sudden fright?

It is possible that a chemical fight-or-flight reaction within the body can induce spasm or constriction of a blood vessel to such a degree that full momentary closure can actually occur. Such closure, followed by complete obstruction of blood flow, can cause the formation of a blood clot. Also, a vivid reaction of fear or terror could induce an abnormal heart rhythm pattern. Both of these situations might cut off the oxygen supply to at least part of the heart.

Anyone having a heart attack would know the warning signs of angina?

No. Not necessarily. There are no absolutes. Sometimes there are no immediate warning signs. Sometimes a heart attack just happens.

Symptoms preceding a coronary can occur over weeks or even months. Angina goes from stable to unstable to angina at rest. Many cardiac patients are warned many times of their heart attack risk. Sometimes they listen, sometimes they don't.

In my experience, those who listen usually can avoid the coronary thrombosis if they seek medical advice and change their lifestyle immediately. Sometimes a cardiologist, seeing serious artery disease and the risk of obstruction and heart attack, will suggest bypass surgery (the rerouting of blood flow through the heart, detouring around the heavily plaqued vessels), but even a quadruple bypass is not a cure for coronary artery disease. It is a stopgap measure unless lifestyle changes accompany the operation.

To repeat, heart disease is an illness riddled with denial. If you don't face the prognosis and if you don't change your lifestyle, congestive heart failure and a coronary thrombosis can become real and imminent possibilities.

Is it possible to have a heart attack without ever having had stable or unstable angina?

Absolutely. Some people have artery disease and don't feel angina pain. A recent study in the *New England Journal of Medicine,* in fact, found an association between mental stress and silent ischemia (oxygen deficiency resulting from constricted or obstructed blood vessels) in people with artery disease. In other words, artery disease coupled with mental stress can produce the antecedents of a heart attack and you may not even know it.

How do I know if my chest pain is angina or a heart attack?

You don't know. It could be neither. It could be any of the other conditions we've discussed in this book. You'll know when your doctor finds out and tells you.

The chest pain of a heart attack can often be the same as that of angina; that's why any chest pain is reason to seek medical attention.

What is the usual pain of a heart attack?

Most often it is described as a heavy, pressing pain in the mid-chest area. It can be dull or sharp. Sometimes it feels like there is a piano sitting on your chest.

It is important to remember that the intensity of the pain does not indicate the severity of the condition. Many people with a chronic angina problem are all too likely to pop some nitroglycerin and not call for help. So it is conceivable that those for whom heart attack chest pain is the greatest may actually be the luckiest, because pain can confront unawareness or denial and possibly produce early enough responsive action.

The pain of a heart attack, like the pain of angina, may not even occur in the chest area. It can be a jaw pain or a back pain; it may or may not be a more intense pain than that of angina. Sweating and dizziness are some more obvious clues that what you are feeling is not angina but potentially a heart attack. If you have these other symptoms and recognize them and take action, consider yourself relatively lucky. Some heart attacks are painless and may remain so until it is too late.

You can have a heart attack and not feel anything?

Yes. This is called a *silent heart attack*. In some cases a person may not know he or she has had a heart attack until the next physical examination. We're not really sure why silent heart attacks occur or why they produce no pain. What we do know is that they seem to be more common in diabetics and that they can predispose you to more serious medical consequences if ignored. A silent heart attack can even be fatal, though it is difficult to know if a fatal heart attack was or was not felt by its victim. In any case, this underscores the importance of early diagnosis and treatment of cardiovascular disease.

You said some people will mistake a heart attack for angina and take nitroglycerin. Does the nitroglycerin work if you're having a heart attack?

Nitroglycerin dilates blood vessels. It does not remove plaque or dissolve clots. During a heart attack, dilating the blood vessels can give very temporary relief to the pain, but it will only rarely—if ever—treat the condition, and believing that nitro *is helping* is therefore dangerous if it delays getting proper care.

Wouldn't I know if it wasn't working?

Logically, yes. If the nitroglycerin isn't working as well or isn't working at all, that is a definite clue that you need immediate medical attention.

Sometimes the symptoms of angina and the early symptoms of a heart attack are only subtly different; yet, most people can detect these differences, at least subliminally. There is something different. There may be a conscious sense of doom, which doesn't usually accompany angina.

The big question is whether you listen to your instincts and increase your chances of survival and full recovery by getting help right away. All too often a person suffering a heart attack is a person who has ignored previous warning signs and who knows he or she is at risk. It's like being caught in the bank vault when the alarm goes off. Do you surrender to the authorities or run away? Dealing instantly with a heart attack cannot only mean the difference between life and cardiac arrest, but the speed at which a coronary *is* treated can mean the difference between a nearly full recovery and permanent cardiac illness with all its limitations.

Why is that?

The chest pain may be the warning sign of an impending heart attack. That is, the complete obstruction may not have yet occurred. Cardiac infarction (heart muscle death) may have just begun or may be about to begin. Every moment you wait could mean the loss of muscle tissue and the decrease of cardiac capacity.

How much time do you usually have before this heart muscle is completely dead?

There is no way to know or for me to estimate. It depends on the location of the clot, the individual involved, and the health of the rest of the heart, as well as the side of the involved area and the prior condition of your cardiac and overall health (whether or not you have diabetes, for example).

Suffice to say that *you* have *no time*. The paramedics may have seconds or minutes or even hours in which to save your life and the life of your heart. But you have no time because there is nothing you can do beyond getting prompt medical assistance. Most people who die of the complications of a coronary thrombosis die within the first three to five hours, and most of them spend the first two hours of their coronary trying to decide whether or not to call for help or whether to take another swig of antacid.

What about aspirin? Doesn't that help dissolve clots?

Recent studies have shown that aspirin, when taken orally *in conjunction* with intravenous doses of other clot-dissolving medicines, can expedite the clot-dissolving process. There is no evidence, however, to suggest that self-administering aspirin is a safe idea. What if it's not a heart attack? What if it's an esophageal rupture with hemorrhaging? An aspirin under those conditions could contribute to your bleeding to death. So you don't want to play doctor with yourself or have someone who's not a doctor play doctor with you. You are in a potentially volatile situation. You don't want to throw water onto a fire until you're sure it's not electrical. I recently heard an interview with a researcher who was part of a study that supported the potential benefits for aspirin in saving lives during coronaries. When asked whether people would benefit from administering it themselves while waiting for medical assistance he agreed, hesitantly. He said, "Yes, but only if they are sure it is a heart attack." And he did not explain how you can be sure you are having a heart attack—because there is no way.

How does a doctor properly dissolve clots?

Clot-dissolving chemicals (the same ones used to treat a pulmonary embolus) are injected directly into the clot. I hesitate to list these life-saving chemicals because by the time anyone reads this, new and more effective ones—or newer more effective methods of using old ones—may be discovered, which can increase your chances of survival, provided you get immediate medical attention.

If blood vessels are contracting because of spasms or other reasons, we may need to use a balloon (a device that is passed through the clogged vessel and widens the vessel so that the clot can pass). Sometimes both clot-dissolving chemicals and a balloon are used in conjunction to reduce the risk of subsequent blood vessel obstruction.

Although a recent government-funded study found that balloon angioplasty procedures have become widely overused, I still think it is safe to say that since the discovery, approval, and use of these technologies, thousands of people who would otherwise have died or been irreparably damaged by a heart attack have been saved and enabled to recover. Thanks to the help of some very brilliant minds, the support of medical research, and probably a little luck, help for the heart attack victim is now most often just a phone call away.

Once the clot is dissolved, are we pretty much out of the woods?

Sometimes, but you don't know and your doctor will not feel you are until about 96 hours have passed. It is in those first 96 hours that additional complications may occur.

What kind of complications?

We must watch for re-forming clots. They can re-form in the same place or a new location and, in either case, need to be dealt with—either by re-treatment, ballooning, or even immediate coronary bypass surgery. The severity of the blood vessel disease underlying the heart attack may necessitate this immediate bypass surgery to prevent another coronary.

Heart rhythm irregularities (including sudden ventricular fibrillation), which can be fatal, can rear their troublesome heads. We must observe these closely and, if necessary, stabilize the heartbeat either with medicines or with electrical equipment.

Pericarditis, which you'll recall is an inflammation of the

lining of the heart, may result as a complication of a heart attack. This can potentially confuse diagnosis because the pericardial pain may alter the patient's description of his or her chest pain. Once diagnosed, this complication usually heals by itself if there are no further complications of the heart attack.

Other potential complications we have to watch for during the first four or five days are congestive heart failure and potential shock, both requiring immediate medical attention.

Again, the sooner you get help upon feeling the chest pain, the less likely you will suffer these complications and the more likely you will be in the right hands if and when they do occur.

What about dead heart muscle tissue resulting from a heart attack?

Sometimes we can do surgical repair to replace dead heart muscle tissue. In fact a recent study at Emory University found a large back muscle—called the latissimus dorsi —very helpful in cardiac repair surgery. This particular muscle is ideal because it is large, because it has ample blood supply, and because the effect on the back of losing part of this muscle seems to be minimal. And, since the muscle comes from inside of the patient's body, we reduce the risk of rejection.

Of course, if, as I will emphasize in the next section, you have acted fast and maintained some degree of calm, this damage may often be minimal.

Part Three
ANSWERING PAIN WITH ACTION

Preparation for and Relaxation During the Most Stressful Moments of Your Life

How does a person prepare for the medical emergency of a chest pain?

It's a very tricky issue. Since many of the illnesses that cause chest pain are preventable by healthy lifestyle habits, it is much saner to prepare yourself *not* to have the medical emergency of a chest pain. On the other hand, it is probably foolish to believe that you have ultimate and absolute control over every aspect of your health. Health is how you choose to live your life and that includes these preparations. And anyway, there is no conflict between these two ideas because probably the most important preparation you can make in order to survive a serious medical emergency is something that will promote health and help prevent this very kind of emergency.

And what preparation is that?

Learning how to relax through deep breathing, muscle relaxation, and meditation. We will deal later with the specifics of implementing relaxation during an actual emergency, but for now understand that relaxation is not a magic pill or formula. It is, I believe, an acquired skill or ability, something you have to learn the way you would learn any exercise or skill. And by learning and developing relaxation for yourself, you will probably greatly reduce your risk of heart disease, ulcers, panic disorder, and many other illnesses that can cause chest pain.

How do I learn these relaxation techniques?

The first thing you need to do is find a doctor who believes in the significance of the mind-body connection and the importance of relaxation and stress reduction and who has some awareness of how it is achieved. Obviously, if your doctor is a type-A, hurry-up-diseased person and seemingly destined for a heart attack of his or her own, it isn't likely you will receive much inspiration in the way of relaxation. Also beware of medical technocrats.

What's a medical technocrat?

Any doctor who places more value in the various wonderful machines and data of medicine than in his or her own eyes, ears, hands, and heart and who believes the lab results before believing your own description of how you feel.

Unfortunately, it is becoming increasingly difficult for a medical student not to become a technocrat. The rigors of medical school are such that humanity and compassion are often learned outside the classroom—if ever. And these days *all* of us in the medical profession tend to get swept away by the wonders of modern technology, because the advances are staggering and potentially life-saving. Yet, they still do not compensate for having a heart doctor without a heart. You want a doctor who is going to see you not as a set of symptoms, oxygen saturations, venous pressures, and preconditions but as a person.

It is true that there is an increasing awareness among everyone in the medical profession that stress is a serious health issue. You are about 100 times as likely to be asked by your physician, "Are you under stress?" today than 20 or 25 years ago. But if the answer is "Yes," as it all too often is, many physicians will simply catalogue this as a medical fact and not talk to you about reducing it. Some physicians believe it is in the realm of psychiatry to deal with stress and anxiety. For some it may be but not necessarily for everyone. Find a doctor who has some suggestions for coping with stress or who is at least concerned about the state of your job, career, marriage, sex life, and self-esteem.

What do you suggest to your own patients?

I do sometimes recommend psychotherapy, but many patients cannot afford it or simply won't go. And even if they do, I don't assume therefore that I, as physician, no longer have any responsibility to help the patient learn relaxation.

For that reason, I also recommend meditation, chanting, hatha-yoga, deep-breathing techniques, and music (preferably something with a smooth, calm, steady rhythm with which your heart can syncopate). If you are religious (I may not need to tell you this), prayer is a most effective stress reducer. Even if you're not religious, praying to some higher consciousness or life force—just the simple act of prayer —can help center you.

What if I'm a devout atheist?

Then I would ask, "Do you believe in poetry?" Because reciting poetry to yourself can be very relaxing. Here's where your preparation comes in, not just for medical emergency but for any emergency or stressful situation. Find a poem, preferably a rather short poem, that relaxes you and memorize it. Or a chant—religious or otherwise —or a prayer. Anything. Even a song such as "Ninety-nine bottles of beer on the wall," if the repetition of that refrain relaxes you.

I like to use images. I'll mentally paint a beautiful landscape. In fact I'll even tell you what it is. It's the view of ocean and wooded mountains from the Santa Barbara Mission. No, I was never a monk there (though sometimes I have wished I was), but, when I was a medical student and the pressures of exams were becoming unbearable, I used to escape by driving up the coast and spending a few hours at the Mission. And now, when I feel anger or fear or any bad stress coming on, I reconstruct the scene—to the tree branch, adobe shingle, cloud and bird, and the one monarch butterfly of this exact moment I remember. I try to hear the soft, natural, unmechanized sounds. For you, it may be a particular place along the ocean, a lake, or a park; it may be a backyard from your childhood or a ski resort from your adulthood.

The point is, your preparation is to find out what relaxes you and keep it handily in the front of your mind.

How else should I be prepared for medical emergency?

If you live alone, I think it's a good idea to have someone call to check on you once a day—like the buddy system when you're learning to swim. The teacher, who cannot possibly ensure the safety of all ten or twenty kids at once, pairs them up into buddies, the idea being that each pair keeps an eye on one another and it is less likely that anyone will drown.

Also, have your doctor's number handy. After you dial 911 and get a paramedic on the way, you may want to have someone call your doctor. If 500 other people in your city decided to have a medical emergency the same night as your chest pain and the paramedics are too busy to get you with their usual promptness, your doctor can possibly find you a private ambulance or some other safe means of getting immediate medical attention.

Should I investigate the various emergency facilities near where I live?

It can't hurt, but I wouldn't emphasize it as part of preparation. When you dial 911, you are giving up your power of choice. You are going to be delivered to wherever the paramedics deliver people from your street (and anyway the most important treatment you may receive may be right inside that ambulance, where many lives and much heart muscle are saved). And who's to say that if you're going to have a chest pain you're going to be at home? You could be across town or on the other side of the world.

Yes, what if I am in Bangkok or Reykjavík?

I suggest to my patients that whenever they arrive in a foreign country they find out from the hotel or from the American embassy what sort of medical emergency facilities are available and how they are quickly accessed if needed. Of course, I also make sure a patient sees me for a physical examination before traveling abroad to reduce the chances of ruining a vacation with a sudden illness.

But if I'm near home I shouldn't worry about where they take me?

I can't tell you what to do. It isn't my nature, and anyway, people listen to suggestion with more seriousness than they listen to ultimatum. Most people I know of who've had medical emergencies—chest pain or otherwise—have turned their lives over to the care and discretion of paramedics, and I have no reason to believe that these people did not receive the best available medical treatment in the timeliest fashion possible.

I have also known a few kind souls who have refused to surrender control and tried to drive themselves to the hospital of their preference. I have known doctors who drove their mothers, fathers, wives, and husbands to the hospital they believed had the best emergency facilities. Even when they do make it in time and can brag about their 85-mile-per-hour automobile adventures, I am still not impressed. Not just because these same heroes could easily have been very sorry or very dead but because it is this very kind of omnipotent stunt, and the struggle for control and power it expresses, which is a major cause of heart disease and a great obstacle to recovery.

If there is one potential benefit to a heart attack or any medical emergency (assuming you survive it in relatively good health), it is that it can, pardon the expression, kick you in the ass. It can knock you off the high horse you might have been riding toward your own early death. If a type A personality is a health risk, humility and a giving-up of complete control can be a life-saving gift. They are, at the very least, steps toward inner freedom. Driving yourself 20 miles to your favorite medical complex is *not* the first step toward such freedom.

Is there anything besides relaxation techniques that I should have on hand while waiting for paramedics?

I've suggested to patients who have a significant risk of cardiac or pulmonary illness to keep some oxygen around.

Oxygen?

Pure oxygen. You can buy a small canister for about 40 or 50 dollars at a medical supplier. If your chest pain is accompanied by shortness of breath, pure oxygen inhaled through an open mask can help you get deep breaths and achieve relaxation. Oxygen can provide a sense of security to some people —to know they're taking some action while waiting— and it cannot hurt.

There are no known side effects to breathing in oxygen?

Very funny. No, if we could all breathe oxygen in its proper ratio instead of the sometimes toxic gas we now call air, we would probably live longer and healthier.

Isn't it dangerous to smoke near pure oxygen?

If you are waiting for paramedics to save you from what may be a heart attack or some respiratory emergency, it is dangerous to smoke, period. In fact, it is insane, which is not to say that many people don't do it. Don't be one of them.

Any other at-home medical equipment I should have?

No, but having you and your family learn CPR can be a lifesaver.

What's CPR?

Cardiopulmonary resuscitation is the artificial maintenance —by something other than the heart—of the heart rate, breathing, aeration, and circulation. It can be done with machines but anyone who has learned how can do it manually as a temporary measure.

Where do my family and I learn CPR?

CPR is taught at many hospitals and as part of community service programs all over the country. Your doctor should be able to recommend a good place to learn this valuable skill.

What about those medical bracelets that list allergies?

If your doctor or you know of any medications you are allergic to or of any conditions, such as diabetes, hyperthyroidism, blood abnormalities, or brain diseases, which might necessitate a modification of medical treatment, it is certainly a good idea to make this information as easily accessible as possible.

The problem I have with medical identification bracelets is that they are jewelry. You can misplace or decide not to wear it. The bracelets are also difficult to update, and your health status is always changing.

So what do you suggest?

Keep the information in your wallet, which is almost always with you and which paramedics are trained to examine if you fall unconscious. One idea is to have your doctor print this data on the back of one of his or her business cards or keep it on a piece of colored, easy-to-identify paper that you can revise as often as necessary. If you have a heart condition of any kind, ask your doctor for a photocopy of your latest EKG and keep that in your wallet as well.

Any other preparations I should make?

Yes. Medical insurance. Choosing the right plan is a book in itself, a book that might have to be revised monthly. You do not want to find yourself with a chest pain and no coverage. Most people I know who do not have medical benefits through their job or union have an emergency policy with

PREPARATION AND RELAXATION

a high deductible; it doesn't usually pay for routine medical visits, but it is there in case hospitalization or surgery ever becomes necessary. Without some kind of insurance, it is even possible that you could be denied medical treatment by some facilities.

Okay, so it happens. My chest feels like the Statue of Liberty is sitting on it. I've called the paramedics and I'm waiting. Every second seems like forever. I'm scared to death. What do I do?

Sit down in the most comfortable chair you can find (don't lie down), take a deep breath, meditate, visualize, pray, think of funny things, and make yourself relax or recite poetry to yourself. Whatever you have previously found helps relax you, do it.

What if I don't know how to meditate? What if I ignored all of your preparatory advice?

Then the first thing you need to do is forget what you did and didn't do. Forget you were ever supposed to learn everything. You did the best you could. You called the paramedics. You'll have plenty of time later, God willing, to make restitution to yourself for your recalcitrance and to get on the right track. Find the most soothing music—in your head or on your hi-fi—and listen. Visualize warmth in your hands and visualize the muscle within your chest contracting and expanding with the same beat as the music (a good reason not to select free-form jazz, modern classical, or any other avant-garde music).

Fear is a crippling emotion. It really can worsen whatever condition is causing the chest pain. Yet fear does not stand a chance against faith. Any kind of faith. Faith in God. Faith in a more abstract concept of a higher intelligence. Faith in medicine (yes, we're not perfect, but we do try awfully hard). Faith in your own inner healing abilities. Fear may also be dealt with through laughter, as proven by Norman Cousins, author of *Anatomy of an Illness.*

What if it is my husband or wife or mother or father who has the chest pain? What can I do to help him or her relax?

Relax yourself! Fear is a communicable disease. Open his or her clothing to allow easy breathing, make him or her as comfortable as possible. Believe that this is an adventure you will both survive. Do not allow the other person's panic to speed up your heartbeat. On the contrary, you must maintain that 70 beats-per-minute concerto until he or she is in harmony with you—play some Mozart or Mendelssohn if it is accessible.

What should I expect when the paramedics arrive?

The paramedics are going to take full control of the situation. They are trained to know what to do, and it is a very good idea to assume that they do in fact know what they're doing. They will ask you whatever it is that they need to know, and you really don't need to offer any other information. The best advice, up front, is to trust them and make a decision to be a follower, not a leader. They are not interested in your theories or diagnosis as to what you're experiencing.

What sort of things do they want to know?

Why did you call?

PREPARATION AND RELAXATION 161

I have a chest pain . . .

Details, we need details. How you describe your pain will, of course, depend on what you are experiencing, but there are some good words to remember that can help communicate and possibly help guide them toward the correct immediate treatment.

What are those key words of pain description?

1. Type of onset:
   Did it come on suddenly, like a flash of lightning?
   Or did it build slowly, like a rumble to a deafening roar?
   Once the pain struck did it dissipate? If so, did it return again? If so, how quickly?
   Or did the pain strike and then fade slowly?
   Or did it strike and maintain its intensity?

2. Pain location:
   Front, back, deep within the chest, outside of the chest, or straight through from front to back?
   Upper chest, lower chest, upper stomach, middle of chest, right side, left side, or all over?
   Does the pain radiate? If so, does it radiate up, down, right, left, up and to the right, down and to the left, or all over?
   Make sure to describe all pains you are aware of, even if they are not all in the chest area!

3. Type of pain:
   Knifing?
   Burning?
   Cramping?
   Ripping?
   Tearing?
   Pressure?

Compression—as though a vise were clamped on your torso?
Crushing—does it feel as though 100 pianos were resting on your chest?
Electric?
Mild ache?

4. Progression since onset:
   Has it gotten worse?
   Gotten better?
   Stayed the same?
   Changed in location or intensity or type?
   Do not be afraid to say it has gotten better or disappeared altogether! Do not be afraid to tell them that the pain is no longer in your chest but is now in your wrist! Tell the truth!

5. Pain responses:
   Is pain relieved by a specific position or motion?
   Is it made worse by a specific position or motion?
   Do positions and motions not have any effect on your pain?
   Does breathing affect pain?
   Does pain affect breathing?

6. Other critical symptoms:
   Shortness of breath?
   Palpitations?
   Nausea?
   Are you hot?
   Are you cold?
   Are you wet?
   Are you hot and wet? (fever)
   Are you cold and wet? (shock)
   Did you have a sudden urge to urinate and/or defecate at the onset of pain? (This is no time for modesty. Your life is at stake!)
   Did you or do you have diarrhea?

What else are the paramedics going to want to know?

How long have you been feeling this pain? Did you take anything for it? Have you taken any medicines within the last four to eight hours (or any pills whose dosage spans a 24-hour period)? Your answer should include coffee or any caffeinated beverage or alcohol. Even cocaine. Your doctor is not going to have you arrested. But if you don't tell the whole truth, he or she may not be able to help you. In fact, there are two people to whom you should never lie: your doctor and your lawyer.

The paramedics will need to know if you've fallen or had an accident within the last few weeks. Tell them, even if it's an embarrassing accident. If you were drunk and tried to rollerskate down a fire escape, the paramedics did not come to criticize your sensibilities. If you were in a fight and lost, no one is here to rank your pugilistic skills. You could have an unknown fractured rib or other bone condition. Help the paramedics help you.

If there is time, they may ask about any preexisting medical conditions. If this information is in your wallet, give it to them. If not, tell them whatever you know.

The paramedics may want the telephone number of your doctor. They may not. The important thing is that you let them concentrate on the most important thing, which is your body and what's going on to cause the chest pain. Try not to distract them in any way. Yield to them. This is why relaxation and the ability to have faith is so vital. Too many people find themselves afraid to trust these strangers who are suddenly in their house, wanting to take over. They waste precious time and emotional energy asking: "What's that?", "Why are you sticking that thing in me?", "Why do I have to lie down?", "Why are you putting that mask on my face?", and so forth. Try to remember that *you* called them. They've come to help. Thank them for coming and then let them do their job.

Okay, wonderful, I'm relaxed. I'm keeping my mouth shut and I'm letting them do their job. Then they carry me into the ambulance, crank up the siren, and scare the hell out of me. What do I do?

First let me tell you what *not* to do. Don't say, "Oh, God, that siren is me. I'm dying!" Most of us are used to hearing a siren and thanking the Lord that it is not coming to get us. When it is, there can be a tendency toward panic and depression, though many people report that the sound of the siren was a sound of reassurance and actually helped relax them.

How do I keep from getting panicked and depressed?

Well, since I've never, knock wood, been in that position, I can only share what I've learned from my patients. Those who did not allow the stress of the situation to dominate them and to compromise their already imperiled health have conveyed a number of experiences. Some of them simply combat fear with irony and humor. Instead of "Oh, God, that siren is me!", their inner voice says something to the effect of: "A fine mess you've gotten me into, Stanley."* Others simply chanted something simple, religious or not. One woman said she repeated to herself: "I'm gonna live, I'm gonna live . . ." until she hypnotized herself into a state of calm. A television writer told me he just imagined that his life was a week-long miniseries and it was only Tuesday. Other people said they approached the unnerving experience as an adventure. They imagined they were children on an amusement park ride. Still others found themselves calmed by focusing on the moment, as though they could see their life through a microscope, frozen in time. Each moment became enormous. And this sensation, strange as it

---

*If you don't understand this reference, rent a Laurel and Hardy movie. They can help teach you the art of laughter.

may seem, gave them a sense of strength and a feeling of confidence that they could overcome whatever illness they had.

What should I expect when I get to emergency?
Action and possibly not words. Remember when you handed your life over to the paramedics? Well, they're going to hand it over to the folks at the emergency room. These people move quickly and deliberately. They often have a lot of people to take care of and not a lot of time. They will often speak sharply and to the point in order to save time and in order to save the lives of you and everyone around you. If they seem rude and unconcerned, believe me, they are not. Measure their concern for you in the concentration on their faces as they get your IV started or take your blood pressure. If someone asks a question you have already answered to the paramedics, answer it anyway.

This is no time to express your distaste for repeating information or your personal critique of the lack of communication in contemporary society. Nor is it the appropriate time to express your opinion about being made to sign an insurance form while you're in such physical peril. I have seen patients blow their stacks when an admitting clerk asked for a signature. Although I agree that it is rather a brutal procedure, anger at such moments is potentially suicidal—and that goes for anger at anyone. Don't start a mental laundry list of all the people—your wife, your husband, mother, father, kids, landlord, tenant, boss, employees—whose misbehavior you may believe has caused your heart attack or ulcer or what-have-you.

Anger is not only one of the most dangerous complications of *whatever* illness or condition caused your chest pain, but it certainly is not going to endear you to the emergency room staff. Remember, they are human beings. They have feelings and they are already under a great deal of pressure.

I'm not saying they're going to neglect you and let you die if you don't shower them with affection. What I'm saying is it can only help to be kind. You don't have to smile through your pain. Just say "Thanks" when someone comes by to change your IV bottle. Try it. You'll win over the hearts of everyone in that emergency room.

But how do I control my anger in that situation?

Since your anger is probably the result of fear, you have to deal with fear. Replace it with faith. You have to believe that these people are going to do whatever is humanly possible to save your life. In all likelihood, they are.

Should I tell a few jokes if I'm up to it?

That's a big *if,* and I'd save most of my comedic repertoire for later. I don't know about all doctors, but when I'm trying to decide which medicine or medicines to use—considering your condition and whatever other drugs you might have in your system—and how much to give you per drop per minute and do this while keeping my peripheral vision constantly watching what the monitors are telling me, the last thing I need at that moment is the next Bob Hope trying out his latest routine. No, on second thought, that is only the second to last thing I need. The *last* thing I need is a patient or the relative of a patient asking me to explain everything I'm doing and compare it with similar procedures on *St. Elsewhere.* Anyone who knows me knows how important I think doctor/patient communication is and yet, when it comes to a medical emergency, that communication has to be nonverbal. It must be an understanding that I am trying to save your life and that that is my expression of love and respect for you, and I'll explain it all to you later—for now I'm too busy trying to make sure there *is* a later.

If I shouldn't ask questions and I shouldn't make jokes, what do I do with all my nervous energy?

Repeat that prayer or poem or chant. Make affirmations to yourself. One of my favorites, for any unpleasant circumstance, is "I deeply and profoundly accept myself in the worst of times." Just keep repeating it. Try to paint that beautiful picture in your mind. Listen for the music. Glance over at that IV flowing into your veins and imagine that it's liquid vitamin L, love, entering you in megadoses.

You said the last thing you, as a doctor, need in the emergency room is a demanding relative. What if I'm the relative and I'm there with my sick wife or husband, how should I behave?

Do whatever you are told by the emergency staff. Stay out of their way, and that goes for your ego as well as your person. Do not instigate anything resembling a power struggle. Show trust in the professionals on whom your friend or relative is relying. Believe me, showing distrust is not going to get better care for your loved one. Show appreciation. But most of all, be supportive and comforting to your wife or husband or whomever. Be optimistic. Here's where some jokes can come in handy.

Remember that we all possess, within us, a tremendous capacity for survival. Sometimes, we just have to get out of our own way or be helped by someone we love to get out of our own way.

I really do believe that everything, even a survived heart attack, can be a learning experience. If it can teach you to change your lifestyle and live longer, what a gift!

In the next section, we'll talk about the lifestyle that promotes cardiovascular health.

The Fifty-Year Cholesterol and Hypertension Plan

Why is it a 50-year plan? Is it going to take me 50 years to get my cholesterol and blood pressure under control?

Of course not. But simply getting cholesterol and blood pressure out of the danger zones is only a small part of cardiovascular health. That's why, in my opinion, health schemes that emphasize the biochemical change without giving equal attention to the accompanying lifestyle and attitudes is a short-term solution at best. Actually, 50 years is just an estimate. The point is that cardiovascular health is not something you acquire and forget. It is an ongoing approach to living. For you, this could be a 60- or 70-year plan. Think of it as the "plan."

Okay, what's the plan?

To begin with, you need a simple understanding of the complex risk factors of the cardiovascular system. They can be narrowed down to two, genetic predisposition and lifestyle.

What is a genetic predisposition?

Some of us are born with congenital heart illness or structural defects. Most are relatively rare and can be dealt with early in life. Other genetic predispositions to heart disease are much harder, if not impossible, to detect. Some people believe that they inherit a certain vulnerability to heart disease. Perhaps many members of their family suffer from —or have died of—heart and/or circulatory problems. The rationale is that, if two people from different families lived identically, one might develop heart disease while the other would not. However, since no such study has ever been conducted, the only congenital illness we know of that predisposes us toward cardiovascular disease would be diabetes.

What does diabetes have to do with heart disease?

Diabetics have trouble metabolizing sugar and fat, which means that a diabetic consuming the same amount of excess saturated fat as a nondiabetic would probably have a greater chance of suffering from blood vessel disease. But that is not a death sentence. The most recent report from the American Diabetes Association found multiple risk factors for diabetics, all of which can potentially be controlled, including insulin dosages themselves. In other words, by ambitiously reducing fat and sugar consumption, the diabetic can probably overcome the risks of that illness.

For most people, I happen to believe that who your parents are has very little to do with your health as an adult. The fact that one or both parents or other relatives suffered from heart disease or coronary thrombosis usually *does not* mean you are destined to the same fate. And the belief that because your parent or parents died at a certain age means you will too is, for the most part, mythology. When a patient despairingly wails to me how Mom and Dad were cut down in their respective primes by coronaries, I always ask, "But what foods did they eat? How much did they drink or smoke? How much exercise did they get? How much stress were they under?" These issues—the way we live our lives while we're here—have the greatest impact on how healthy our hearts will be.

What specifically do you mean when you say "the way we live our lives"?

Diet, exercise, emotional status and attitudes (including the negatives, cynicism, hostility, and impatience), and vices (which include excess use of over-the-counter medicines and other drugs). I used to approach all these factors in cardiovascular health as separate issues. I no longer do. I believe now that they are all interrelated under the category of lifestyle.

How are they interrelated?

Each factor can affect each other factor. Therefore, to deal with each as an isolated issue or to concentrate on one to the exclusion of the others is a big mistake.

You cannot, for example, separate diet from exercise. Exercise has a direct effect on nutrition. How much activity we engage in each day helps define our metabolism, which is the efficiency with which our bodies use what we eat. Exercise not only uses calories, it also tells our body not to store so much fat. Exercise has also been found to help suppress the appetite, and, in my own experience and the experiences of some of my patients, vigorous daily activity can influence a desire for the right kind of food selection. At the same time, nutrition affects exercise. What we eat can determine how much we want to and in fact *can* exercise. Excess refined sugars and refined carbohydrates can often engender lassitude and lethargy and turn us into couch potatoes.

Exercise and our emotions are also interlinked. Vigorous

activity can relieve depression, anger, and stress. A sedentary life can magnify boredom and cause depression.

Our emotional makeup has a direct effect not only on how much we are likely to exercise but also on what food choices we are likely to make and on the habits—good and bad—that we will engage in. At the same time, what we eat, smoke, drink, and otherwise consume or fool around with is bound to help shape our emotional state.

Cigarette smoking and other harmful habits and addictions can also affect and be affected by all the other factors. The same is true of nutrition, including food allergies, which we are continually finding out can have a radical effect on the emotions and on overall health.

What this all adds up to is that, if, for example, you deal simply with diet and neglect to consider the other choices in your life, it isn't likely you're going to make a lasting impact on cardiac health and longevity. If you cope with emotional stress by eating yourself into a state of sedation, you could very well be relaxing yourself into a coronary. If you start a vigorous exercise program and don't quit smoking, you're taking a big risk with your immediate health. If you eat sanely, exercise regularly, quit bad habits, and learn to relax but still avoid intimacy, you might still be putting yourself at a long-term health risk.

Where do we begin?

You begin with a commitment, a commitment to yourself—an affirmation or love for yourself—that you love your life enough to want to do your part toward cardiovascular health. "Sure," patients sometimes tell me, "so I can get hit by a truck and die anyway." But the fact is that most Americans still die of unnecessary illness, and most of these illnesses are probably a direct result of the way in which they lived their lives. A lifestyle enhancing cardiovascular health can also greatly reduce the risk of cancer and many other potentially life-shortening illnesses.

Okay, I'm committed. I want to live to a hundred. Now what?

Now we'll find out just how committed you are. First, let's take a look at your destructive habits and addictions. Some recent studies have suggested that one drink per day is not harmful—and may actually be beneficial—to cardiovascular health. The most up-to-date report I've seen on the subject found that women who had three drinks per week seemed to reduce coronaries by 30%, whereas those women who consumed between three and nine drinks per week *increased* their coronary risk by that same 30%. I'm not yet fully convinced of any of this but, so as not to seem too inflexible and conservative, let's say that between zero and one drink per day is probably fine. And, if you're going to have a drink, why not make it one light beer (one without cobalt as a foam stabilizer)—just in case the theory is wrong. Just a thought, not an ultimatum. But no more than one drink—and remember that one drink per day does not mean abstinence Monday through Friday and then seven martinis on Saturday night.

What if I need more than one drink?

Need is an interesting word. If you mean you cannot relax without two or three drinks, then perhaps you need to learn how to relax. Hatha-yoga, meditation, deep breathing, taking a walk, listening to Mozart, and group therapy are all ways to learn how to relax. If you seriously have a physical need to drink, then you may want to answer the 20 questions that Alcoholics Anonymous asks a prospective member.

As for cigarette smoking, I don't care what Philip Morris III says. As far as I'm concerned, tobacco smoking is no longer a controversial subject. The American Lung Association, the American Heart Association, and the Surgeon General have been warning Americans about the dangers of smoking for years. I will assume that their message has not eluded you and will therefore refrain from repeating it in detail. Obviously the only healthy intake of burning tobacco is zero and this includes passive smoking.

Passive smoking?

That means breathing in the cigarette smoke generated by someone else. Recent studies have found a significant cardiac and pulmonary risk to people who live with a heavy cigarette smoker or who work in an environment heavily polluted with the smoke of burning tobacco.

What if I am a smoker, how do I quit?

There are many methods. As increasing numbers of Americans make the decision to quit and quit-smoking clinics continue to be a growth industry, there may be many more. Surgeon General C. Everett Koop has recently declared cigarette smoking not only to be an addiction but also perhaps the most difficult addiction to overcome, which suggests that something beyond willpower is required. Quit-smoking methods include counseling, acupuncture, nicotine chewing gum, hypnosis, behavior modification therapy, and self-help literature. And if I left any out I did not do so to suggest that it was any less effective than any other. In fact there is no absolute proof as to the effectiveness of any single method, though the study in the *Journal of the American Medical Association* that I mentioned earlier reported that, regardless of the overall quitting method, one factor seemed to increase greatly the chances of success.

What factor was that?

Human contact. Smokers who had the most frequent face-to-face contact with a counselor or some other human support system developed the most long-term motivation to keep from lighting up. This would probably hold true with regard to any substance addiction, including caffeine. Why not start your own support group of caffeine addicts trying to quit this harmful drug? There may also be a biochemical answer to help conquering the cigarette addiction. A drug, known generically as clonidine, that is used commonly to treat high blood pressure may actually help break the smoking addiction. You may want to ask your doctor about it, if cigarettes are standing in the way of your cardiovascular health.

And you say I have to give up caffeine as well?

Yes. Caffeine can initiate irregular heart rhythms, raise cholesterol, stimulate anxiety, panic, and hurry-up disease. And we're not just talking about coffee. Caffeine is commonly found (and sometimes hidden) in colas and other soft drinks, teas, chocolate, hot chocolate products, and many over-the-counter medicines (especially those which boast of being "extra strength" and "fast acting").

Okay, I'm clean. One drink maximum per day. No cigarettes or caffeine or other harmful drugs. Now what?

Well, the most important thing for you to understand now that you've shaken off the various monkeys of habit and addiction is to watch out for perfectionism.

Perfectionism?

Another significant contributing factor to heart disease. The need to be perfect—considering that you are an imperfect creature living in an extremely imperfect world—can lead to frustration, anger, and the kind of stress that can potentially damage your heart as much as any of those nasty substances.

How do I avoid perfectionism?

Say that you've made an honest commitment to quit smoking and avoid passive smoke. You find yourself on an airplane one row from the smoking section, and the plane is full and you cannot get another seat. Just relax, breathe in the smoke-polluted air, and know that one airplane ride of passive smoke is not going to shorten your life, but that the anger, frustration, and stress of your situation could, if not contained, have a much greater impact on cardiovascular health.

Say that you've given up caffeine and discover that the fruit punch you're drinking has been spiked with some caffeinated beverage. Forget it, relax, and get a glass of water.

I could go on.

Don't. Okay, so I'm clean and I'm also only human and proud of it. Now what?

Take a walk. A vigorous walk. Or any other constant vigorous exercise—with your doctor's approval. Anything that increases your breathing and heart rate for a minimum of 20 to 30 minutes.

The reason I mention exercise before diet and stress management is that I believe exercise has a more direct effect on those other two factors than vice versa. If you don't know what to do, where to begin in your quest for cardiovascular health and if cholesterol and saturated fat and complex carbohydrates seem, well, complex, and the idea of reducing the stresses in your life seems impossible, all you have to do to get the ball rolling is take a walk.

I usually recommend one mile per day for starters, once I've established with an EKG or treadmill test that the patient can handle this without risk. Nonstop. Not walking the dog and stopping at every tree and fire hydrant.

Just the simple act of taking a vigorous one-mile walk

every day can help the other areas of your lifestyle. I have seen patients begin this kind of activity and then discover they no longer crave the same high-fat, low-nutrient diet they'd been feeding themselves for so many years. They tell me walking helps reduce stress. I tell them it lowers their blood pressure. Patients tell me that when they feel themselves getting tense, they take a walk and cool off.

There are many other benefits to a daily cardiovascular workout. Countless studies have found that people who live sedentary lives do not live as long or as healthfully as active people, regardless of sex, age, ethnicity, or political party. A recent study I just read found that physical activity had an *inverse* relationship to heart disease in middle-aged and elderly men (and probably would have concluded similarly for any age group of either sex).

This means that if you work in a sedentary job (which most people in our current economy do) then you have to find a way to be active before or after work.

What if I work all day and the streets of my city are not safe to walk at night?

A real problem for some people, because in some parts of some cities it isn't even safe to walk the streets during the day. Also, those who live in cold climates or in very hot or humid climates face a similar problem. Indoor shopping malls are often a good alternative. Most are safe and climate-controlled. Of course, you can't stop to shop until you've finished your mile or two. If there are no malls or if they don't open early or late enough to accommodate your schedule, you can always join a health club that has treadmills or get a treadmill for your home. Treadmills usually have built-in odometers so that you can keep track of your workout and know when you've completed your mile —or two.

In a mall, how do I know if I've walked a mile or two?

Use an attachable odometer. They cost about 10 or 20 bucks and fit right on your belt. They will keep track of speed and distance. I know people who've been mall-walking for years. Some people have walking clubs. They meet early in the morning, when the mall is uncrowded, and walk. They walk vigorously, but they're also able to make it a social experience—which leads us into another diversion, further confirming how interrelated all the components of a health-promoting lifestyle are.

And what might that be?

The importance of social experiences, of feeling a sense of purpose and belonging. Of having friendships and loving relationships, of being a vital part of this world. Loneliness is a major health issue. The human organism can be amazingly resilient. I believe that that resilience owes itself largely to the state of mind of its occupant. Later in this chapter I'll suggest a plan of vitamin and mineral insurance. Make no mistake about it, there is one vitamin we need far and away more than any of the others. That's vitamin L for love. If we are both loving and loved, we not only have more to live for but we also vastly increase our chances of living longer.

So start walking and do it with other people if you can. There is no reason exercise can't be fun. In fact, fun is as important to cardiovascular health as fiber, which I'll talk about shortly.

What about other kinds of exercise? What about sports?

Anything that gets that heart muscle pumping faster— continuously for about 20 to 30 minutes—is great, providing your doctor judges it not to be too strenuous. I don't happen to recommend sports because they're not for everyone, and it's important to stress that cardiovascular health *is* for everyone—everyone who wants it, anyway. I have patients who thrive on tennis or cycling or jogging. I have seen patients, men and women, take up boxing at their local gym (with protective headgear, I assume). Whatever turns you on. I have also had patients who said they used to love tennis but found it got too stressful, with partners being late or empty courts hard to find or arguments about the score.

What if you don't have time to exercise?

Don't have time? Think of it as the other way around. If you don't exercise, you may not have time because you probably won't live as long as if you do. We can always make time. People who live a hectic life—and to some degree you really have to ask yourself how much of it is really necessary and how healthy is it—can always get an exercise bicycle and plant it in front of the TV. If you have time to watch the news or three innings of a baseball game, you have enough time to give your heart muscle some much-needed attention. Of course, you have to be careful to set the tension properly and to work yourself up gradually. For me, though, riding a stationary bike (or walking on a treadmill, for that matter) and staring at the same four walls—or at the same news anchorperson's face—is boring with a capital ZZZ. I like to walk with my eyes as well as my legs. Then walking becomes an adventure and not a drudgery.

Traveling is another reason why I make walking my exercise of choice. I've had more than one friend and patient complain about trying to find a health spa in order to swim that mile or pump that iron while on a business trip or an emergency. If you're a walker, you can explore the place you're visiting and get your daily cardiovascular workout at the same time. And that's not all.

Wait, don't tell me. Walking enhances your sex life?

No, that wasn't what I was going to say, but now that you brought it up, I suppose it could. I mean, to begin with, that a vigorous walk is relaxing and, if done for a long enough stretch of time (doctor permitting), it can induce the release of those wonderful endorphins into the bloodstream, and, certainly, anything that enhances cardiovascular health is a must for a robust sex life. Finally, perhaps most important of all, if you take that walk with the one you love—or with the one you want to love—well, I mean, you can slow down a little bit . . . after the first mile.

But sex wasn't what was on your mind when you said "That's not all." What was?

Walking can also be a great cure for constipation.

Why is that?

Gravity and muscular abdominal wall motion massage the intestines and bowels. Walking an hour a day and drinking ten to fourteen glasses of purified water is the simplest solution for this and many other gastrointestinal disorders which, as you now know, can cause chest pain and mask the symptoms of heart disease. By the way, walking is also an important part of the treatment of many kinds of arthritis (another potential cause of chest pain), as well as osteoporosis.

But there is one final benefit from being of a mind-set that walking is good, that it's fun, and that it can extend your life.

What's that?

When I pull into a parking lot to park my car, I no longer have to confront the stress and anger of competing with twenty other drivers for those good spots. If the place looks even remotely crowded, I look for the farthest space I can find. I might even pull out of the lot and park three blocks away, knowing that I'm giving myself a treat: a walk. Maybe it's a busy day. Maybe I wouldn't have had time for my walk or for all of it. What a lucky guy. Suddenly all those other drivers in the parking lot have done me a favor.

The same goes for crowded elevators. I look for the stairs, assuming I'm not going to the 42nd floor. Climbing stairs can be a great workout and much more pleasant than sharing an elevator with some stressed-out people angrily eyeing the elevator panel as every button lights up. Of course, you'll want to check with your doctor before climbing any stairs and always make sure you haven't walked into a flight of fire stairs that lock from inside.

What if I can't walk? What if I'm in a wheelchair?

Do aerobics.

In a wheelchair?

Sure. You can get a fully aerobic workout just by using the upper part of your body for 20 minutes. Here are some examples:

1. Extend the arms all the way out and twirl them in tight six-inch circles. Twirl them forward. Then twirl backward. Start out slowly, then speed up. Do it as fast as you can and keep it up for as long as you can.
2. Swing your arms up and down—jumping jacks without the jumping.
3. Lift the shoulders up, around, and down, in a circle. Do it faster and faster, then maintain your fastest speed for as long as you can.

CHOLESTEROL AND HYPERTENSION PLAN 181

4. Swing the arms front and back, up and down, as you would if you were shaking out a blanket (or shake out a blanket for 20 minutes).
5. Learn the violin or viola.
6. And here's my favorite: with a piece of uncooked linguini, conduct the Brahms C-minor Symphony (or the orchestral selection of your choice).

If you want to get really ambitious, hold two- or three-pound weights in your hands and try these exercises. They're ideal not only if you're in a wheelchair but if you sprain an ankle or a knee or anything that keeps you off your feet, even temporarily. If you, God forbid, ever wind up in traction and you feel up to a cardiovascular workout, sing.

Sing?

That's right. People who sing or vocalize regularly can help increase their cardiovascular strength and endurance.

What if you have a really terrible voice?

Sing in the shower. Take singing lessons. Sing along with Frank Sinatra or Sarah Vaughan and keep the volume up high so that no one hears you.

Okay, I'm walking and conducting and singing. Now what do I eat?

Well, that's easy. You're a person, right? So you wouldn't eat dog food. Dog food is for dogs. Cat food is for cats. And junk food is for junk. You're not junk, and if you think you are then we need to talk about self-esteem because that is also a health issue. Low self-esteem may have a profound effect on our ability to recover from illnesses such as heart disease and, possibly, to reduce the risk of getting sick. It is almost a medical proverb now that self-esteem—our opinion of ourselves—has a direct effect on immunity. And self-esteem has just as much, if not more, impact on the choices we make in our lives, such as what to eat. Do we deserve the best? Do we deserve what (many of us already know) is best *for us?* If you need to make a drastic change in lifestyle in order to stay healthy, do you have the belief in yourself? I say all of this because so many are aware of what a health-promoting lifestyle means. "Easier said than done," they tell me. And they're right. And without self-esteem it can be even harder.

So what do I do if I have low self-esteem?

Well, as a cardiologist and not a psychiatrist, I tell my own patients to put the body in motion and let the mind and spirit follow. Pretend you really love yourself and behave like you do. After a while, you might begin to believe it. The paradox is that you cannot live a health-promoting lifestyle until you develop high regard and respect for yourself, but in many ways you can't develop that self-respect until you're living the life that makes you smile at the mirror.

Now I'm ready. What's the diet?

I'm not a dietitian. Think of me as a voice trainer.

We're back to singing again?

No. Not that kind of voice training. I'm going to try and train the voice in your head, the one that makes choices for you, over whether to exercise when you'd really rather watch someone else do it on the Wide World of Sports. The voice that, after the initial explosion of anger, decides whether to hold onto the hostility and rage or whether to let it go, for the sake of your health.

That's the same voice that tells you what to eat. Some

people think that voice is hopelessly capricious and cannot be trained. That's why diet books make the bestseller list. The diet book is supposed to be a restraining order on that inner voice. Unfortunately the voice will only stay restrained for so long. That's why so many people's bookshelves are lined with so many different diet books. If any of them worked, why would there be so many?

How do I begin to train my voice?

Since arteriosclerosis is probably the most significant cause of heart disease, let's start training it to make the kind of choices that can reduce the chances of your arteries becoming sludged and clogged.

Are we talking low cholesterol?

Yes and no. First, let me explain exactly what cholesterol is. There are a number of different substances all known as cholesterol. Two in particular are of major concern to your health. They are high-density lipoproteins *(HDL)* and low-density lipoproteins *(LDL)*.

LDL are the bad guys. They carry fat cells to the arteries, where they combine with calcium and other substances to form plaque and cause atherosclerosis and plugs. HDL are the good guys. They don't get nearly as much publicity, probably for the same reason that murderers get more press than people who work for the Peace Corps. HDL is an essential fatty substance that helps transport fat and LDL *away from the arteries* to the liver, where bile takes over and dumps this harmful cholesterol into the intestines.

So the good cholesterol gets rid of the bad cholesterol?

Precisely. The word cholesterol has generically come to mean LDL cholesterol, which Surgeon General Koop recently reported is far too great a part of the American diet.

But a new study just released from Johns Hopkins University may begin to bring HDL cholesterol into the limelight. This research suggests that a shortage of HDL is a more significant factor in raising the risk of coronary artery disease than excesses of LDL cholesterol. This means that many diets and so-called cholesterol "cures" may not be nearly as effective in curbing heart disease as believed.

Before you tell us what we can't eat, let's start with what we can eat. Where do we get good-guy cholesterol?

Not from eating. The only known way to elevate this essential fat is through exercise. Another great reason to take a walk and make that walk a part of your daily life. There are, however, foods you can eat that can *lower* the LDL cholesterol.

What are they?

Monounsaturated fats, eicosapentanoic acid (EPA), and fiber.
 Monounsaturated fats are olive oil and canola oil (a.k.a. rapeseed oil). And they must be consumed in moderate amounts (about one tablespoon per day, on salads or cereals) because, like all fats, they are high in calories and like all fats, most of their calories will remain as fat in your body and can turn to body fat. And body fat is one of the contributing factors in raised bad-guy cholesterol.

So one tablespoon of olive oil on my salad each day is good for me, but more than that is bad for me?

Yes. Also, you cannot heat the oil or it will turn from a monounsaturated fat to a saturated fat, the kind you don't want to eat.

You mean I can't fry chicken in olive oil?

Not if you're trying to lower or maintain a low LDL cholesterol level. Heating oil oxidizes it into sludge material. This, by the way, goes for polyunsaturated oils like corn oil and vegetable oil. That commercial that showed your typical American family frying chicken in vegetable oil and grinning about how the chicken has no cholesterol is grossly misleading. The only frying I would consider safe is an *occasional* Chinese stir-fry. But we'll get to food preparation a little later.

What about eating polyunsaturated oils cold?

It is true that they do not raise LDL cholesterol, but they don't lower it either. And, like monounsaturated oils, if eaten in excessive quantities, they can become excess body fat, which can elevate LDL cholesterol. Excess polyunsaturated oils may also present other, noncardiac health risks. So, if you have a choice between mono and polyunsaturated fats, let the voice in your head choose the olive oil. Oh, and beware of the label "vegetable oil" and vegetable oil products that contain tropical oils. Coconut oil and palm kernel oil are sometimes labeled as part of vegetable oil, suggesting that, like corn oil, they are polyunsaturated. They are not. They are as volatile to your LDL cholesterol level as beef lard. Read labels. Also, any time you see the word partially or fully hydrogenized, you're reading about a saturated fat. Reject it. Anyway, by the time this voice-training session is over, your voice will be poised to reject most of those processed foods that are largely the cause of the Surgeon General's latest findings.

What about EPA?

Eicosapentanoic acid, according to the most recent studies, not only lowers LDL cholesterol, it also seems to reduce the viscosity of blood, which better enables oxygenated blood to pass through already-narrowed blood vessels. The most up-to-date studies have even found a possible link between this essential fatty acid and *raised* HDL cholesterol. EPA may also be helpful in fighting arthritis, psoriasis, and other inflammations, in lower blood pressure, and raising the body's immunity.

Where do I get EPA?

Fish, fish, and more fish. Deep-water fish to be exact. The best sources seem to be mackerel, salmon, trout, bluefish, cod, flounder, haddock, herring, shrimp, and swordfish.

What about heating this EPA?

Good question. Obviously, you don't want to eat raw fish. That can be very dangerous. Fish eaten raw can cause hepatitis, vibrio infection, and a number of parasite-related illnesses. Heating EPA does *not* convert it to saturated fat, just as heating an olive or an ear of corn does not convert the fat within it into hydrogenated or saturated fat. Of course, deep frying fish does make it into an LDL monster. Steaming or poaching fish seem to be the best ways to cook it.

Are you suggesting fish every night?

Not for everyone. If you love fish the way I do, yes, absolutely. If not, take your time developing a taste for it. Eating should be enjoyable as well as healthful. In fact, in order for it to be healthful I believe it *must* be enjoyable, because pleasure is a big part of maintaining health. Fish is probably the best protein source for the prevention of heart disease, but there are others. Skinless white-meat chicken is another. White-meat turkey isn't bad once in a while.

If you choose not to eat fish every night, you may want to talk to your doctor about EPA fish oil capsules. They are available as a supplement, like a vitamin pill, and seem to have the same positive effects. Use them cautiously, though. There is no established dosage as yet, and they should probably not be taken with aspirin, because both substances are blood-thinning agents and can cause excessive bleeding in some people.

What about fiber?

There's a real advertising buzzword. Fiber. You're supposed to get loads of it and, according to television advertising, the best way to get fiber is from cold breakfast cereal. Well, it certainly isn't a *bad* way to get some fiber into your digestive system, but it sure as heck isn't the only way and probably not the best way. Many of these products contain excess sugar and sodium, and some bran and granola cereals are often coated with tropical oils, which elevate the very same LDL cholesterol the fiber in the cereal is supposed to reduce.

How does fiber lower LDL cholesterol?

Not all fiber does. There are two kinds: water-soluble and water-insoluble. Water-soluble fiber absorbs fat in the blood system and in the intestines and then carries those fats out via the liver into the stool. Anything that removes lipid molecules from your body is going to lower LDL cholesterol.

Where do I get this water-soluble fiber?

Oat bran, apples, bananas, pears, melons, peaches, pineapple, raisins, figs, prunes, papayas, kiwis, berries, artichokes, asparagus, beans, broccoli, brussels sprouts, celery, carrots, cauliflower, cabbage, corn (popped or on the cob), parsley, parsnips, peas, peppers, potatoes, spinach, turnips, and yams, to name a few.

Make sure, by the way, that you clean and then eat all

edible skins of these various foods, and take your juicemaker to the pawn shop because when you juice a fruit or vegetable you are removing its most nutritious part—the part containing the fiber.

What about the other kind of fiber?

Water-insoluble fiber also prevents the reabsorption of bile acids and cholesterol from the small intestines and slows the absorption of sugar, which may actually help elevate HDL cholesterol.

Water-insoluble fiber also works as a kind of broom through the stomach and colon. It helps digestion, helps prevent constipation, inflammation of the intestines, diverticulosis, and cancer of the colon. It may also help in preventing many other gastrointestinal disorders, the kind that can cause chest pain and mimic heart disease, and in that sense water-insoluble fiber is important to the heart.

Where do I get it?

As it turns out, if you're getting your water-soluble fiber from oat bran, beans, carrots, peas, potatoes, or yams, then you're probably already consuming sufficient water-insoluble fiber. That's because all these foods are great sources of both kinds of fiber. Other water-insoluble fiber foods are wheat bran, barley, kasha (buckwheat), and brown rice.

What about all these new drugs that are supposed to lower cholesterol? Should I be using them?

Cholesterol-lowering drugs are expensive and have potential side effects. They are usually used as a last resort, if nothing else works. If your doctor prescribes them for you, he or she has decided that the expense and potential side effects are outweighed by the dangers of your high cholesterol. Of course, if you haven't been completely honest —if you've said that you've stopped spreading butter on your morning toast and you really haven't—then perhaps what you need more than medicine is a little honesty. In my own practice I often prescribe psyllium husk, a natural anticholesterol agent, before putting a patient on any of the medicines. The only side effects of psyllium husk or any other natural source of fiber are *good* side effects. By building a diet on a foundation of fiber you will, for example, also be satisfying your body's need for complex carbohydrates.

What are complex carbohydrates?

The only kind on my table. I won't bore you with too many details of a subject we have all been inundated with, but perhaps I can shed some new light.

Carbohydrates are the foods that give us energy. There are two kinds of carbohydrates: refined and complex. Each energizes in a different way. Refined carbohydrates— white sugar, white flour, and all of their thousands of prepackaged derivatives—pack a wallop. Almost everyone knows if you eat a candy bar you can experience a sudden burst of energy, sometimes even a semi-euphoria. As your blood sugar rises, this feeling can last anywhere from 20 minutes to an hour or two. When your blood sugar plummets, you're drained, fatigued, even depressed. I liken these refined sugars and carbohydrates to an unreliable friend or lover. They're great for a while. They make promises of lasting bliss. Then they drop you like yesterday's newspaper and leave you in shock and despondency.

Complex carbohydrates are your loyal friend. They metabolize slowly, giving a steady, realistic, nonhyped flow of energy. Complex carbohydrates may not pack a wallop, but they do pack a wealth of lasting energy, as well as vitamins, minerals, and other nutrients. So let's get that voice within talking about fresh fruits, vegetables, and whole grains.

What specifically are the cardiac benefits of complex carbohydrates?

Several. To begin with, the highs and lows of white sugar and white flour (also known as white paste for what it turns into during digestion) can speed up and slow down your heart rate, putting added strain on the pumping muscle. In fact, if you consume large amounts of white sugar and then exercise, you can induce chest pain, tachycardia, fatigue, and panic disorder. The refined sugar molecule, if consumed in excess, can also be converted into a triglyceride, which is one of the components of arteriosclerotic plaque. Furthermore, obesity is a major contributing factor to arterial and heart disease, and refined carbohydrates are probably one of the major causes of obesity in America.

Why is that?

There are several reasons. Because refined sugars and carbohydrates take you on that blood-sugar rollercoaster, they promote, rather than satisfy, hunger. People on this rollercoaster may tend to eat these foods again whenever a letdown occurs—which can be quite often. The little or no nutrition they offer may promote a physiological hunger for what the body is not getting. I have often said, and I'm not the only one, that thousands of Americans are simultaneously overweight and malnourished.

Foods high in refined sugars and carbohydrates are usually also high in sodium, which not only elevates blood pressure and greatly increases the risk of heart disease but can also create an intense thirst many people mistake for hunger, which they keep feeding. Remember that potato chip company that boasted about their product: "Bet you can't eat just one"? Well, they've changed their advertisements but not the recipe of their product.

Finally, these refined sugars and carbohydrates deliver an artificial, overstated flavor. Like elevator music turned way up, it fills up time and space but offers no really rich experience. Complex carbohydrates are like Mozart. When you're finished, you feel you've really eaten something.

And what does obesity have to do with cardiovascular health?

Plenty. Obese people are at a much greater risk for heart disease and heart attack (not to mention a myriad of other illnesses). To begin with, body fat itself is one of the major causes of high cholesterol and arterial disease. Excess body weight also puts a tremendous strain on the heart muscles and circulatory system but does not strengthen the heart equivalently the way exercise does.

Where does obesity begin? How much should I weigh?

For women, figure about 100 pounds up to five feet tall, then add five pounds for every additional inch of height. For men, figure about 110 pounds up to five feet tall, then add six pounds for every additional inch of height. Consider yourself obese if you are 10% to 15% overweight.

But if you allow yourself a lifestyle promoting cardiovascular health, you aren't likely to maintain much excess weight. Body fat is mostly the result of dietary fat. In other words, fat on your fork turns to (or should I say *remains as*) fat in your body. About 97% of the fat you eat, in fact, remains as fat in your body. Complex carbohydrates, on the other hand, only turn to fat if eaten in excess.

Having said all that, I must add that an occasional piece of cheesecake or ice cream cone—or eating a piece of your own birthday cake once a year—is not going to cause arteriosclerosis. Thank God, because perfectionism, as I said earlier, can definitely increase your cholesterol and your risk of heart disease.

Why is that?

Well, emotional stress, which is almost a certain side effect of perfectionism, elevates LDL cholesterol. I have seen patients who exercised regularly and whose diets were admirable yet whose blood cholesterol levels were alarmingly high. In almost all cases, these people were under intense anxiety or depression.

So if you do have that occasional ice cream bar, don't multiply the cholesterol with guilt and anxiety. It is important, however, to make that piece of cheesecake or that ice cream cone the exception and to acknowledge to yourself at the time that it is an exception—a guiltless but cautious exception. If you already suffer from severe arterial disease or from diabetes, then you may not be able to afford such a luxury.

What I see as dangerous is to eat a cheeseburger with french fries and actually believe this is a nutritious, healthy, and well-balanced meal. Or eating a hunk of frosted carrot cake or a plate of deep-fried zucchini and calling it a vegetable. Let's get that voice inside your head to be honest.

Aside from preventing obesity, what else do complex carbohydrates offer in the way of cardiovascular health?

They promote exercise and stabilize emotions, both examples of the interdependency of all the components of a healthy cardiovascular lifestyle.

Complex carbohydrates are our body's most nutrient-dense and reliable sources of energy. They are, therefore, foods that fuel our ability to exercise. In other words, how are you going to walk your mile or two or three when you're lying on your back with a white paste hangover? Just as exercise can affect diet, diet can affect exercise.

Diet can also affect your emotions. Refined sugars and carbohydrates promote stressful highs—and can even bring on panic disorder in some people—as well as potentially agonizing lows. Complex carbohydrates encourage emotional stability and, since they promote weight control, can enhance self-worth.

All that from something that grows in the ground?

Isn't it amazing? But don't assume that because a food is natural and untampered with that it necessarily promotes cardiovascular health. Avocados, for example, are very high in calories and should therefore be eaten in small quantities. Coconut is a fruit, yet its meat contains a saturated fat that can raise LDL cholesterol. Actually, the word "natural" has no legal definition anyway, enabling any box or bag of pseudo food (with the names of 28-syllable chemicals on its panel) to claim to be "all natural." Dairy products such as whole milk, cheese, butter, and eggs can truly be natural or unprocessed and still, over time, plug arteries. As with most elements of health and medicine, there are few absolutes.

Knowing that, what do I eat?

Let's start with what you drink. Water. And lots of it. Drink 10 to 14 glasses per day of purified water. Water is the main ingredient in our blood supply. Healthy cardiovascular circulation is dependent on a constant fresh supply of fluid.

And you say purified?

I use reverse osmosis at home and at the office. From what I have read, this particular system is the best way to remove bacteria and parasites without allowing them to settle and procreate on the fibers of the filter itself, as in activated charcoal. Some bottled waters are good, others are not so good. There are thousands of bottled water companies throughout the country and several publications that attempt to rate these waters. I try to use bottled water when I am traveling. When it is not available, I cross my fingers, relax, and drink up.

What do I eat in between my 14 glasses of water per day?

That must be up to you and that voice we're trying to train. But if I can remember, I'll tell you what I had for breakfast this morning and what I'm going to have for lunch this afternoon and dinner tonight.

Breakfast was a bowl of hot Kashi with blackberries. For lunch I'll probably have a shrimp and crab salad with a tablespoon of olive oil and a dessert of watermelon. For dinner, with any luck, I'll poach a salmon, steam two greens and a yellow vegetable, and then cheat on a fat-free frozen yogurt.

The way you choose to *cook* your food has as much to do with the prevention of heart disease as your food selection. Vegetables are best when eaten raw, lightly steamed, or microwaved. I like to broil or poach my deep-water fish without grease. Even *broiling* in oils and butter can take a wonderful food and erase its benefits and then some. Of course, there will be times when you are invited to dinner at someone's house and everything on their table has been cooked—or even saturated—in butter. Sometimes in a restaurant, even if you tell the waitress to cook your salmon without butter, it will still come to the table dripping with those tiny beads of cholesterol.

What should I do?

Well, in a restaurant, you could send it back. That would certainly be an exercise in self-esteem and a devotion to cardiovascular health. But sometimes it is not possible. You

CHOLESTEROL AND HYPERTENSION PLAN 195

may not have time. And in the case of the dinner party, you may not want to complain about the food in any way.

So what do I do?

Relax and eat the fish. Don't take life so seriously. The anxiety you might create by delaying your hurried meal or by upsetting the social circumstances is far more dangerous to your heart than *one* piece of salmon prepared with butter. So is the anxiety you might inflict upon yourself about eating that one piece of butter-drenched fish (and you don't have to eat the whole thing).

You see, cardiovascular health is very much a matter of choices, decisions, and approaches to situations as they arise in your life. If you miss exercising one day because of a crisis or a deadline in your work or the demands of family or friends, don't panic. Relax. If you exercise every day, missing one day is not going to shorten your life, but anxiety and panic will. If the demands of family and friends seem to be compromising your health, just remember that simply having family and friends is a major part of good quality health for your heart and every other part of your body. If you arrive on your vacation in Tahiti and you discover you or your spouse forgot to pack your vitamins, relax and enjoy your vacation. If you've been taking the daily insurance of vitamin and mineral supplements, your cell fibers aren't going to start deteriorating in the course of a few weeks.

What vitamins and minerals should I be taking to reduce my chances of heart disease?

Well, I cannot categorically state that any one particular vitamin or mineral is, in and of itself, a substance that directly prevents heart disease. But I strongly believe that just as the components of a health-promoting lifestyle are interrelated, so is the physiology of health and of illness. General health promotes cardiovascular health. If, for example, your immunity is strong, you are less likely to suffer a viral infection of the heart. I will, therefore, simply spell out my recommendations for the vitamin and mineral insurance. These recommendations are meant only to ensure an adequate amount of all the necessary vitamins and minerals. If you choose to build your daily diet around complex carbohydrates, deep-water fish, and monounsaturated fats, you will be getting most of your daily requirements. But you never know. Not every flower of broccoli has the same amount of vitamin A as every other flower. And anyway, who wants to go around measuring the nutrient composition of every food you eat? Talk about boring. So eat from the garden and then make sure from the multi-tab. (If you're receiving chemotherapy, get your doctor's specific approval for vitamins.)

LOOK FOR A MULTI-TAB WITH:

10,000 to 25,000 IUs of *betacarotene**

15 to 100 milligrams (mgs) of *thiamine (B_1)*

30 to 50 mgs of *riboflavin (B_2)*

30 to 50 mgs of *niacin (B_3)*

50 to 250 mgs of *pantothenic acid (B_5)*

25 to 50 mgs of *pyridoxine (B_6)*

100 to 400 micrograms (mcgs) of *cobalamin (B_{12})*

50 mcgs of *biotin*

1000 mgs of *choline*

100 mgs of *inositol*

40 mgs of *PABA*

400 mcgs of *folic acid*

---

*Betacarotene is the precursor to vitamin A. By taking it in the precursor form, you eliminate any risk of vitamin A toxicity.

400 IUs of *vitamin D*

100 to 400 IUs of *vitamin E*

THEN LOOK FOR A SEPARATE DAILY TABLET GIVING YOU:

1000 to 2000 mgs of *vitamin C**

LOOK FOR A MULTI-MINERAL WITH:

2 mgs of *copper*

100 to 150 mcgs of *chromium*

10 to 15 mgs of *manganese*

15 mgs of *zinc* (preferably as *picolinate*)

500 to 750 mgs of *magnesium* †

10 to 15 mgs of *manganese* †

100 mcgs of *selenium* †

THEN LOOK FOR SEPARATE TABLETS OF:

1500 mgs of *calcium*

Take *iron* only if your doctor diagnoses a deficiency or anemia and prescribes this mineral.

There are also some more controversial supplements available that may be helpful in preventing heart disease. I mentioned EPA fish oil capsules already, and so let me just remind you that it is better to get your daily dosage of EPA from the fish itself—just as it is better to get betacarotene from a carrot or vitamin E from spinach. But, if you're a determined vegetarian and you are serious about lowering cholesterol and reducing the risk of heart disease, you may

---

*Remember, if you have stomach ulcers or gastrointestinal illness, you should probably choose to take vitamin C in the nonacid form.

†You may or may not be able to find these dosages of these minerals in a multi-mineral tablet; if not, look for separate tablets or multis that get close.

want to ask your doctor about EPA fish oil supplements. A doctor's supervision is important because there is no official dosage for EPA capsules. Activated charcoal is also controversial, but early reports are that it seems to lower cholesterol and it is now available in supplement form though there is no official dosage, and so it must be taken under the supervision of a doctor. Finally, there is an amino acid called L-carnitine.

Amino acid? Don't you get those from protein?

Yes. But L-carnitine seems to be plentiful only in red meat, which we want to choose not to eat since (with the possible exception of flank steak) red meat is high in saturated fat. But L-carnitine is pretty important to your heart. It seems to help in the contractile strength of the heart muscle. In fact, if you recall from the section on cardiomyopathy, deficiencies of L-carnitine have been linked to cardiomyopathy in some people. There are no known side effects of supplementary L-carnitine and the FDA has even approved supplemental dosages of this amino acid. So choose deep-water fish and take between 500 and 3000 milligrams of L-carnitine. (Make sure you take L-carnitine and not DL-carnitine, which is potentially toxic.)

What about the rest of your recommendations? Are they according to the FDA daily requirements?

No. In my opinion, many of the FDA's so-called daily requirements are far too low. The FDA, for example, still recommends 60 milligrams of vitamin C for an adult male, while your neighborhood zoo is probably giving five times that much to their monkeys. No, I'm not saying we're all a bunch of monkeys, but we are both mammals with similar anatomies (even if monkeys are smarter than we are) and we weigh about the same. Excess vitamin C is painlessly excreted from the body. So what's the harm in making sure that we are getting enough? You would have to eat an entire bushel of oranges in order to consume as much vitamin C each day as I believe your body needs. And vitamin D has very few food sources that I would consider part of a healthy heart diet.

The truth is that there are no absolutely empirical studies about vitamins and minerals. That's because, thank God, we don't do experiments with live human beings. What medicine attempts to do is to study the results of the way people choose to live. Based upon this information we draw conclusions. At the moment, I believe (as I have for quite some time) those studies that have pointed to vitamin and mineral supplements as important in the maintenance of health. Not as a substitute for health-promoting food choices, not as something to chase down junk food with as a placebo of rationalization, but more as a hedge against the imperfections of life. In my opinion, since there is little, if any, risk involved with the dosages I have suggested, I have yet to be convinced otherwise.

Aren't all of those vitamins kind of expensive?

So might seem a diet of deep-water fish, including shellfish, fresh fruits and vegetables, and olive oil. But, relatively speaking, they are extraordinarily *in*expensive. Liberally estimating, let's say one year's supply of vitamin and mineral insurance costs $1,000. Isn't that the cost of about one day in the hospital? That's not counting loss of wages from work either. The expense of a seafood diet can be annihilated by one heart operation. In fact, the total cost of cardiovascular disease in 1987 was estimated by the American Heart Association to be in the neighborhood of $85 billion, which is not to suggest that such medical treatments that may often be life-saving are not worth the cost.

But if you want to talk economics, be thrifty. Spend as

much money as you have to not to get sick. Buy that fresh produce from the freshest source. Buy the sweetest apples, the crispest lettuce. Pay as much as you have to in order to get the tastiest fresh fish, the leanest chicken, the best cold-pressed virgin olive oil. After all, you want to enjoy what you eat. We're not talking austerity. We're talking health!

What about sodium? You mentioned earlier that a deficiency of sodium can cause problems in the heart's electrical system. How do you make sure you're getting enough?

Unless you are on an extremely low-calorie diet, it is virtually impossible to develop a sodium deficiency. And there is no reason to be on a diet of less than 1,000 calories, which is dangerous for a number of other reasons, including the risk of malnutrition and heart and other muscle protein loss. Almost all foods naturally contain at least some sodium. If you eat 1,000 to 2,000 calories per day, you're going to get enough sodium without adding salt during cooking or at the table and without eating high-sodium junk food (your average fast-food cheeseburger contains as much as twice your daily sodium needs). Too much salt can cause fluid retention within the circulatory system, elevating blood pressure and increasing the risk of heart disease.

Isn't food rather bland without salt?

Myth, myth, myth. There are countless seasonings that enhance flavor without increasing bodily sodium levels. Some examples are garlic, onions, thyme, oregano, dill, basil, and jalapeño peppers. Jalapeños, incidentally, have been found to increase food metabolism and thus help maintain a healthy weight. Of course, if you have any esophageal or stomach or intestinal illnesses, you may want to avoid these and other spices.

So if I cut back on salt, I can control my blood pressure?

Yes, but salt consumption is not the only lifestyle habit you'll want to change in order to help control blood pressure. Anxiety, anger, rage, and other emotional stresses can cause blood vessel contraction and have a profound effect on blood pressure. I recently read about an experiment done back around the turn of the century in which a researcher attempted to prove that large daily amounts of garlic would *lower* blood pressure. (Bear with me, this story *does* actually relate to emotions and hypertension.) Anyway, this doctor had a bunch of people eat who-knows-how-much raw garlic every day and, after a very short time, found that the blood pressure of virtually everyone went way down. Was it some ingenious enzyme in the garlic? Was it garlic's effect on the body's metabolism? No. As it turned out, the breath of the subjects was so putrid from all that raw garlic that family members kept their distance, and that seemed to be what lowered their blood pressure.

Well, anyway, I hope your close relationships are not causing you or anyone you love to have hypertension. Intimacy is part of cardiovascular health. That includes an ability to communicate with those close and not-so-close to you, as well as the amount of vitamin L you're giving and receiving.

When is the best time of the day to take this vitamin?

Vitamin L? Anytime. All the time. You cannot overdose!

What about the others?

With food and water. Remember, any pill taken without water can get stuck in the esophagus and cause irritation or ulceration. Nutritional supplements, taken without food, can upset the stomach. It is also probably best to spread them out over the course of the day. Take your vitamin in the morning, your mineral with lunch, and whatever else there is with dinner. That's what I do most of the time. But if the day ahead of me promises to be a minefield of uncertainty, I will usually take everything with breakfast so that I don't have to worry about it the rest of the day. And if I forget to do that, I try not to worry about it (the only vitamin I can't do without for more than a few hours is vitamin L). Going one day without nutritional supplements is no big deal. This philosophy should not, however, be applied to prescription medicines.

Why not?

It really depends on the medicine and what it is supposed to be treating. As a general rule, if your doctor writes out a prescription for you, it is of the utmost importance that you follow it. I only bring this up because of some rather startling findings that thousands of people die needlessly each year simply because they failed to take their prescribed heart medicine.

Now, I'm no chemo hypeman. For years I've been urging my patients and listeners to be sobering in their approach to the wonderful world of modern chemistry. I believe there are far too many people using and abusing far too many substances—mostly legal ones. There are probably more antihistamine junkies in America than heroin addicts. As I mentioned before, many over-the-counter medicines are spiked with caffeine (usually to enhance the speed of the drug), a substance we know to be the enemy of cardiovascular health. Weight-loss drugs, like phenylpropanolamine (PPA) and its related products, can also speed up your heart to a dangerous—and at the very *least* horribly uncomfortable—rate. But this is not to suggest that all drugs are bad or that they are all potentially harmful to your heart. There are many medications that can save your life and help prevent heart disease.

A sober approach to drugs means knowing that every medicine has a side effect, and that it is always possible that the side effect can be more harmful than the medicinal benefit. Many drugs are known to deplete or block the body's absorption of much-needed nutrients. A sober approach means finding out from your doctor why he or she is prescribing a given drug and what are the known and potential side effects of the drug (including nutrient depletion and absorption blockage) and to have your doctor reevaluate the benefit/risk ratio of the drug about every three months. I always tell my patients to bring with them any bottles of pills they are steadily taking. If nothing else, I sometimes discover that the patient has been accidentally taking his wife's Premarin. But caution and a wary eye for drugs must be accompanied by a deep respect for their potential utility. Modern chemistry does save and prolong lives. It also kills people. I have no idea which it has done more of but I do know one thing: A better awareness and understanding and a more active participation on the part of the patient could increase the number of saved and prolonged lives and greatly reduce the number of unnecessary deaths.

Anything else I need to know about the prevention of heart disease?

Yes. Lots and lots and lots of things. What I have given you are the basics, the rudimentary beginnings, but the training of your inner voice is an ongoing lifelong exercise. The half-life of a medical fact is sometimes as brief as two weeks. Although I (and most of the rest of the medical profession) have no reason to suspect that issues such as the connection between LDL cholesterol and arteriosclerosis will be disproven next year, that is not to deny that much of what I have reported may be overshadowed by some new insight within a few years. What I hope I have provided here is a basis on which to synthesize everything you already know and everything you will learn about yourself in the future. It is not the end of your voice training. It is the beginning.

What about someone married to a heart disease candidate? How does one pass along the word to him or her?

That is a very large and difficult and potentially painful question for many people. Once you begin to take cardiovascular health and longevity seriously and get that voice in your head talking sense, it may seem only natural that the people you love should follow your lead. If you're going to live to your optimum potential, you want them around to keep you company. Suffering through the illness of someone you love is probably the next worst thing to your own illness. For some people it is even more horrendous than being sick.

Unfortunately, we are limited in the influence we may have over other people. There is a self-help group called Al-Anon for the wives, husbands, lovers, and other family members of alcoholics. The group is not designed to instruct people on how to get and keep the alcoholic sober. That is considered to be a very sick and fruitless—if loving—waste of time. The alcoholic will quit when he or she is ready, if ever. The Al-Anon members focus rather on their own lives: living physically and/or emotionally with an alcoholic. When you talk about a person at risk for heart disease —though alcoholics certainly fall into that catagory—it is fair to say that you are likely to at least be dealing with a sober and somewhat rational person. Yet you still cannot enforce your will on another person. I should know. Believe me. I wouldn't still be a doctor if I didn't have a deep respect and love for most of my patients. Yet as hard as I try with some of them, they do not listen or at least they don't follow my medical advice to lose weight, to lower cholesterol, to reduce sodium, to exercise every day, to make time for relaxation. And, I have discovered, trying to control someone else not only does not work, it is also hazardous to your health.

Isn't there something I can do to prevent someone I love from having a heart attack?

I try to give medical advice not as a command but as a loving suggestion, sometimes a concerned imploring. I believe that most people will not respond at all to an order. An insistence that they quit smoking will often result in an increase in their poisonous sucking. I cannot say that I myself do not tend to resent and therefore rebel against anyone who might try to dictate how I should live. What I try to do is state the facts as I see them and set an example by practicing the kind of lifestyle choices I would suggest for my patients and for my readers.

People are an impressionistic species. Watch a small child imitate you or another adult or child. Look at the influence of television and the rest of pop culture on the way we dress, speak, and eat. If doctors ever got control of Madison Avenue and were somehow able to foster a health-promoting lifestyle with the same creative zeal that Coke and Pepsi and McDonald's are promoted to the public, we might reduce heart disease in America by a staggering amount. Since that isn't likely to ever happen, we must be satisfied to set an example in our own small, quiet way and hope that those we love might be inspired.

Those of us who have made a commitment to health and who've begun to train our inner voices must be very careful not to become fanatical bores. Most people have encountered at least one dinner party guest who not only turns away the high-fat dessert but then proceeds to explain why, to the dismay of the host and other guests. That same inner voice that can literally save and prolong and enhance the quality of your life can—if it gets hold of your mouth

—alienate you in a social situation or even in your personal life.

Yet it is important not to hoard your health. A concern for the health of our world and everyone in it is something I cherish very deeply and consider a very important part of my life. I try to participate actively in the ongoing debate and, to the best of my ability and the time constraints of my life, the actual fight to preserve and clean up our environment, to protect our lungs and ultimately our hearts from the dangers of water and air pollution, and to insist upon clear and understandable—and unambiguous—labeling of food products so that consumers who care about health are able to make the kinds of choices they mean to. With the rising cost of medicine and medical insurance, it is not only spiritual but also good economic policy to do whatever you can to promote your own health and the health of those around you, because when they get sick, ultimately your premiums go up too.

We are, in many respects, a nation of sick people. Yet there is hope, lots of hope.

Such as?

The intolerance to cigarette smoking. An entire airline disallowing that virulent addiction from polluting the enclosed cabins of its airplanes.

The fact that the food industry in the past few years has so ambitiously targeted health-conscious consumers with claims about low sodium, all natural, low cholesterol, no cholesterol, less calories, less sugar, and more fiber. Although I abhor the deceptiveness of some food industry claims, the fact that they are even making these claims tells me that people want health for themselves and their families and that people are responding to their doctors and to the Surgeon General and the American Heart Association. The food industry, like any industry, survives only by providing a product that people want. Restaurants have begun to join the health bandwagon as well, offering meals with the American Heart Association seal of approval attached. And although I may find some of the American Heart Association's criteria too liberal, it is (pardon the pun) *heartening* to realize that so many people take them seriously.

Ultimately, the most meaningful thing you can do for anyone, sick or well, stubborn or flexible, is to love him or her. If anything can convince someone to do what is necessary to try to prevent heart disease, it is the power of love.

Here, to leave you with, are some tips I try to get my patients' and my own inner voice to espouse:

TIP ONE:

Make a commitment to cardiovascular health.

TIP TWO:

Make a choice for freedom from destructive habits and addictions, including perfectionism.

TIP THREE:

Take a walk or do the aerobic exercise of your choice every day.

TIP FOUR:

Get your LDL cholesterol below 100 and your HDL cholesterol above 50 by following my other tips.

TIP FIVE:

Don't eat more than 5% of your daily calories as saturated fat. Don't fry food.

TIP SIX:

Make the vast majority of fat consumption from monounsaturated sources. Don't eat more than 15% to 20% of your daily calories as any kind of fat.

TIP SEVEN:

Choose complex, not refined, carbohydrates and make them 60% to 70% of your calories.

TIP EIGHT:

Get most of your protein from deep-water fish. You need only about four to five ounces of protein each day. (If you're a vegetarian, make nonfat dairy and plant sources of protein your staples and consider EPA as a supplement.)

TIP NINE:

Do not cook with salt or add salt at the table; choose nonsodium seasonings and spices; and choose unprocessed foods that have not been saturated with sodium.

TIP TEN:

Drink 10 to 14 glasses of purified water each day.

TIP ELEVEN:

Enjoy your food along with the rest of your life, and spice it up without salt.

TIP TWELVE:

Make sure that you are getting all your needed nutrients by taking vitamin and mineral supplements.

TIP THIRTEEN:

Don't let superstition cause you stress.

TIP FOURTEEN:

Reduce stresses of all kinds through hatha-yoga, meditation, Mozart, stress reduction music (or Duke Ellington or any sounds that relax you), vacations, and deep breathing.

TIP FIFTEEN:

Laugh whenever you can and don't be afraid to cry.

TIP SIXTEEN:

Always take a sober look at the medications in your life. With your doctor's input, weigh the risk/benefit ratio, and never assume that any medication or drug therapy is permanent and not subject to alteration.

TIP SEVENTEEN:

Do not risk your own health trying to control someone else's. Instead, set an example.

TIP EIGHTEEN:

Pass the word, but do it gently (buy this book for your friends).

TIP NINETEEN:

Do what you can to make the world a healthier place, but not at the expense of your own health.

TIP TWENTY:

Take megadoses of vitamin L.

BEYOND LATIN: THE GLOSSARY

ACHALASIA: Loss of nerve tissue functioning for unknown reasons.

AMPHETAMINES: Drugs that stimulate the central nervous system.

ANGINA PECTORIS: An illness that produces pain when the heart cannot meet its own oxygen needs.

ANGIOPLASTY BALLOON: A device which is passed through the nearly closed blood vessel, widening its diameter.

ANTITHROMBOTIC: A medicine designed to prevent blood platelet clotting.

AORTITIS: An inflammation of the inside lining of the aorta.

ARRHYTHMIA: Any abnormal rhythm of the heart.

ARTERIES: Blood vessels that deliver fresh oxygenated blood throughout the body.

ARTERIOLES: Small arteries.

ARTERIOSCLEROSIS: Hardening of the arteries.

ATHEROSCLEROSIS: Degeneration of an artery caused by the constant deposits of fat, cholesterol, fibrin (a blood-clotting material), cellular waste products, and calcium.

AUTOIMMUNE DISORDER: An illness in which, for unknown reasons, the immune system turns against its own body rather than against outside invaders.

BETACAROTENE: The precursor to vitamin A (the dietary substance from which our bodies derive vitamin A) found in all yellow and green vegetables and a wide variety of other foods.

212 GLOSSARY

BILE: A digestive enzyme produced in the liver.

BRADYCARDIA: A dangerously slow heart rhythm often of less than 60 bpm.

BRONCHOSCOPY: A look into the lung with a scope.

BURSITIS: An inflammation of a bursa, a lining that, if unimpaired, allows ligaments or tendons to move without friction.

CAPILLARIES: Small arteries.

CARDIAC ARREST: The heart stops beating.

CARDIOMYOPATHY: Any illness specific to a heart muscle.

CHANCRE: An ulceration (usually caused by syphilis).

CHOLELITHIASIS: The medical name for gallstones.

COLLAGEN DISEASE: Connective tissue disease.

CORTISONE: A painkiller or antiinflammatory substance commonly used against inflammatory diseases such as arthritis; it is a natural hormone produced by the body.

COSTAL CARTILAGES: The cartilages attaching the ribs to the sternum.

COSTOCHONDRITIS: Inflammation of the costal cartilages.

CRUCIFEROUS VEGETABLES: Those of the cabbage family.

CT SCAN: A.k.a. cat scan, a computerized diagnostic imaging technique.

DIABETES MELLITUS: Sugar-related diabetes.

DIFFUSE PAIN: Pain in no specific location.

DIURETICS: Medicines used to reduce body fluid and to lower blood pressure.

DUODENUM: The first part of the small intestine.

ECHOCARDIOGRAM: A sound-wave reading of the heart.

ELECTROCARDIOGRAM (EKG): A medical procedure that tests the electrical activity in the heart.

EMPHYSEMA: A disease of obstructed air flow in the lungs with loss of elasticity of fiber.

EMPYEMIA: Collection of puss that cannot drain and that can cause gangrene.

EPA: Eicosapentanoic acid—a fatty acid found in deep cold-water fish.
EPIGASTRIUM: The upper abdominal area, just below the sternum.
FEBRILE ILLNESS: Any illness producing temperature elevation.
FIBRILLATION: Dangerously uncoordinated contractions of the heart muscle, causing heartbeats so irregular that they are difficult to measure.
FLUTTER: Irregular heartbeats as fast as 300 bpm.
FREE RADICALS: Broken bits of molecules missing an electron.
GALLSTONES: Solidified deposits of bile and cholesterol, usually within the gallbladder.
GASTRIN: A gastric enzyme in the blood.
GASTRITIS: An inflammation of the stomach.
GASTROESOPHAGEAL REFLUX: Hydrochloric acid escaping the stomach and burning the esophagus (a.k.a. reflux esophagitis, heartburn).
HCL: Hydrocholoric acid (stomach acid).
HDL: High-density lipoproteins ("good guy" cholesterol).
HEMOGLOBIN-CARRYING MOLECULE: The chemical in the blood that transports oxygen.
HEMOLYSIS: Blood cell wall breakage.
HYPERTENSION: High blood pressure.
HYPERTHYROIDISM: An overactive thyroid gland that produces excess hormones.
IDIOPATHIC: Not-yet-fully-understood; of unknown cause.
INFERIOR VENA CAVA: The major vein returning blood to the cardiac pulmonary system.
INTERCOSTAL: Between the ribs.
INTRINSIC FACTOR: A chemical produced in the stomach cells necessary for the absorption of vitamin B_{12}.
IONS: Electrically charged atoms.
ISCHEMIC HEART: A heart lacking enough oxygen for its own cell processes per unit of time and contraction.

JAUNDICE: Yellowing of the skin and whites of the eyes, lassitude, and loss of appetite caused by the inappropriate collection of bile within the blood system.

LDL: Low-density lipoproteins ("bad guy" cholesterol).

LIPID: Fat.

LITHOTRIPSY: Shock-wave treatment to dissolve deposits such as gallstones.

LYMPHOMA: Tumor of the lymphatic system.

MEDIASTINUM: The space between the lungs and the heart.

METASTASIZED TUMORS: Tumors spread throughout the body.

MYOCARDIAL INFARCTION: The death of an area of the heart muscle, resulting from a reduced blood supply to that area.

MYOCARDITIS: Inflammation of the heart muscle.

MYOSITIS: Any muscle inflammation.

NEURITIS: An inflammation of a nerve or nerves.

NONSTEROIDAL: Any antiinflammatory medication other than cortisone, which is a substance being pharmaceutically prescribed.

OSTEOPOROSIS: A condition wherein the bones become decalcified and brittle.

PERICARDIAL EFFUSION: A fluid collection—such as bleeding—between the lining of the heart and the heart itself.

PERICARDITIS: Inflammation of the heart lining.

PERICARDIUM: The lining of the heart.

PERISTALSIS: The contraction of the muscle cells such as those of the esophagus.

PLAQUE: A plaster-like substance that hardens arteries and can fully obstruct them.

PLEURA: The lining of the lungs.

PLEURISY: An inflammation of the pleura.

PLEURITIC PAIN: Sudden sharp or grating chest pain usually worsened with each breath and accompanied by shortness of breath, because of an inflamed pleural lining.

POLYCYTHEMIA: Excessive platelets and red blood cells.

GLOSSARY

PNEUMOTHORAX: Free air that gets into the pleural cavity —the area between the lining of the chest wall and the lining of the lung.

POSTERIUM: The rear of the mediastinum.

POSTHERPETIC NEURITIS (HERPES): A nerve complication of shingles.

PROLAPSE: Push backwards.

PROSTAGLANDINS: Hormones, some of which are essential to the maintenance of the stomach's integrity.

PSYCHOSOMATIC: Describing a disorder caused by or influenced by the emotional state of the patient.

PULMONARY ARTERIOGRAPHY: A dye study of the pulmonary blood vessels.

PULMONARY EMBOLUS: A clot somewhere within the lung.

PURKINJE FIBERS: The "electric wires" of the heart that bring the signal to the muscle cells, orchestrating coordination of the contractions.

REFLUX: A flowing backwards contrary to the normal direction.

REFLUX ESOPHAGITIS: Heartburn, or inflamed lining of the esophagus.

SARCOMAS: Tumors of the muscular system.

SEPSIS: General infection throughout the body, once called blood poisoning.

SILENT HEART ATTACK: A coronary producing no symptoms.

SINUS NODE: The heart's natural pacemaker.

SPLENECTOMY: Surgical removal of the spleen.

STERNUM: Breastbone.

SUBSTERNAL: Below the breastbone.

SYSTEMIC ILLNESS: An illness affecting different parts of the body at the same time.

TACHYCARDIA: Regular or sometimes irregular rapid heartbeats of 130 or more beats per minute.

TAMPONADE: Collection of fluid in the pericardial sac that constricts the heart.

VALVE REGURGITATION: Leakage backwards of blood through the heart valves.

VASCULAR: Blood vessel.

VEINS: Blood vessels that return deoxygenated and waste-filled products of metabolism to the heart.

VENULES: Small veins.

WEDGE PRESSURE: The blood pressure within the heart itself.

XIPHOID PROCESS: The very bottom tip of the sternum.

RESOURCES

Blackwell, JN, Castell, DO; "Esophageal Chest Pain: A Point of View." *GUT,* 25 (1984) 1.

Braunwald, E, Hillis, LD; "A thorough Review of Miocardial Ischemia." *The New England Journal of Medicine,* 296 (1977) 971.

Braunwald, E. P.; *Textbook of Cardiovascular Medicine, 2nd Edition.* Saunders Company.

Brensike, JF, Levy, RI, and Kelsey, SF, et al; "Results of the Nhlbi Type II Coronary Intervention Study." *Circulation,* 296 (1984) 313.

Buja, LM, Willerson, JT; "Clinicopathalogic Correlates of Acute Ischemic Heart Disease Syndrome." *American Journal of Cardiology,* 47 (1981) 343.

Cohen, JN, et al; "Effect of Vasodilator on Mortality." *The New England Journal of Medicine,* 3 (1986) 1547.

Dec, GW, Palacios, IF, Fallon, JT, et al; "Active Myocarditis in the Spectrum of Acute Dilated Cardiomyopathies: Clinical Features of Histologic Correlates and Clinical Outcome." *The New England Journal of Medicine,* 312 (1985) 885.

Gillum, RF; "Idiopathic Cardiomyopathy in the United States, 1970–1982." *American Heart Journal,* 111 (1986) 752.

Guiton, AC; *Cardiac Output and its Regulation.* Saunders Company, 1963.

Hogan, MJ, Dacy, MD; "Cholesterol." *Mayo Clinic Health Letter,* 6 (1988) 1.

Johnson, RA, Palacios, IF; "Dilated Cardiomyopathies of the Adult." *The New England Journal of Medicine,* 307 (1982) 1051.

Kannel, WB, Feinleib, M; "Natural History of Angina Pectoris in the Framingham Study." *American Journal of Cardiology,* 29 (1972) 154.

Leaf, A, Weber, PC; "Cardiovascular Effects of n-3 Fatty Acids." *The New England Journal of Medicine,* 318 (1988) 549.

Maseri, A, L-Abbate, A, Baroldi, G, et al; "Coronary Vasospasms as a Possible Cause of Myocardial Infarction." *The New England Journal of Medicine,* 299 (1978) 1271.

McDonnel, PJ, Mann, RB, Buckley, BH; "Involvement of the Heart by Malignant Lymphomas." *Cancer,* 49 (1982) 944.

Rankin, JS, Newman, JR, Califf, RM, et al; "Clinical Characteristics and Current Management of Medically Unstable Angina." *Annals of Surgery,* 200 (1984) 457.

Regan, TJ; "Alcoholic Cardiomyopathy." *Prog Cardiovascular Disease,* 27 (1984) 141.

Reyes, MP, Lerner, AM; "Coxsackie myocarditis." *Prog Cardiovascular Disease,* 27 (1985) 373.

Schneider, RR, Seckler, SG; "Evaluation of Acute Chest Pain." *Med Clinic North America,* 65 (1981) 53.

Shabetai, R; *The Pericardium.* New York, Grune & Stratton, 1980.

Sleisenger, MH, Fordtran, JS; *Gastrointestinal Disease, 4th Edition.* W.B. Saunders Company, 1987.

Snyder, DW; "Mitral Valve Prolapse." *Postgraduate Medicine,* 77 (1985) 281.

Truett, J, Cornfield, J, Kannel, WB; "A Multivariate Analysis of the Risk of Coronary Heart Disease in Framingham." *Journal of Chronic Disease,* 20 (1967) 511.

Trust, JB; *Best and Taylor's Physiological Basis of Medical Practice,* Williams and Wilkens, Co., 1985.

Willerson, JT, Hillis, LD, Winniford, M, et al; "Speculation Regarding Mechanisms Responsible for Acute Ischemic Heart Disease Syndromes." *Journal of the American College of Cardiology,* 8 (1986) 254.

Wyngaarden, J, Smith, L; *Cecil Textbook of Medicine.* W.B. Saunders Company, 1988.

———; "Atrial Fibrillation in Coronary Artery Disease." *American Journal of Cardiology,* 61 (1988) 714.

———; "Mental Stress as a Cause of Silent Myocardial Ischemia." *The New England Journal of Medicine,* 318 (1988) 1005.

RECOMMENDED READING

Biermann, June, and Barbara Toohey. *The Diabetic's Book.* Los Angeles: Tarcher, 1981.
Burns, David D. *Feeling Good, The New Mood Therapy.* New York: New American Library, 1980.
Complete Home Medical Guide. Columbia University Medical School.
Cousins, Norman. *Anatomy of an Illness as Perceived by the Patient: Reflections on Healing and Regeneration.* New York: Bantam, 1981.
Any other book by Norman Cousins.
Dufty, William. *Sugar Blues.* Philadelphia: Chilton Book Company, 1975.
Eater's Choice: A Food Lover's Guide to Lower Cholesterol. Washington, D.C.: The Center For Science in the Public Interest.
Gold, Mark S. *Good News About Depression.* Knightstown, Ind.: Bookmark Books, Inc., 1986.
Lappe, Frances M. *Diet for a Small Planet.* 10th Anniversary Edition. New York: Ballantine, 1982.
Pelletier, Ken. *Mind as Healer, Mind as Slayer.*
Piscatella, Joe. *Choices For a Healthy Heart.* Workman.
Piscatella, Joe. *Don't Eat Your Heart Out Cookbook.*
The Best of Broadway or any other sing-along book.
Anything by Mark Twain, James Thurber, Italo Calvino, Neil Simon, Oscar Wilde, Philip Roth, Bill Cosby, Gary Larson, or any other humorist (who are we to say what's funny to you?).

INDEX

Abscess, Pulmonary 52–54
Affirmations 166–167
AIDS 27, 56
Al-Anon 204
Alcohol consumption 14, 30, 31, 56, 77, 117, 137, 172
Acoholics Anonymous 172, 204
Allergies 14, 76, 89–90, 158, 171
  Panic attack related 89
Anemia 18, 41, 103, 197
Anger. *See* Emotions, High-impact.
Angina 98–113, 141–142
  Causes 99–106, 115
  Diagnosis 106–108, 143
  Pain patterns 107, 142
  Treatment 108–113
Angioplasty balloon 112, 145–146
Antacids 17–18, 28
Aeortic aneurism 68–71
  Pain patterns 69
Arrhythmias 103–104, 114–118, 146, 190
Arteriosclerosis 69, 100–101, 105, 115, 140–142, 191–192, 203
Arthritis 75–77, 179
Atherosclerosis. *See* Artereosclerosis
Attitude, Change of. *See* Stress, Reduction

Back strain 81
Bacterial endocarditis 136

Barrett's esophagus 18–19, 27
Behavior. *See* Lifestyle
Belching 19–22
Blood clotting 47, 140, 145–146
Blood pooling 47
Blood pressure 138. *See also* Hypertension
Bulimics 23
Bursitis 78, 80
Bypass surgery. *See* Cardiac bypass surgery

Caffeine 117, 174, 202. *See also* Diet, Modifying
Campylbacter pyloris 31
Cancer
  Gallbladder 45
  Lifestyle and 171
  Lung 63–66
  Pancreatic 41–42
  Psychological aspect 86
  Stomach 38
Carbohydrates
  Complex 189–193, 207
  Refined 190–193, 207
Cardiac bypass surgery 109–110, 113, 141
Cardiomyopathy 137–138, 198
Cardiovascular disease, Cost 199
Cardiovascular system 97–98, 168–171
  Risk factors in 169–171
  Commitment to health regarding 171–172, 191–209

221

INDEX

Cholesterol 69, 70, 140, 183–189, 203, 207
  How to lower 109, 184–189
Cigarette smoking 30, 41, 51, 58, 63, 76, 83, 84, 102, 113, 157, 171, 172–173, 206
  How to stop 84, 173–174
Cocaine 83, 84, 105, 117
Colitis, Ulcerative 63
Cooking methods, Healthy 194–195
Coronary. *See* Heart attack
Costochondritis 73–75
CPR techniques 157–158

Denial 2, 3, 7, 141
Depression 41, 58, 91–93, 192
Diabetes mellitus 44, 169, 192
Diagnosis, Responding to 5, 15, 18
  Self diagnosis 4, 28
Diet, Modifying your 1, 14–16, 21, 170
  Angina 105, 110, 113
  Arrythmias 116, 117
  Arthritis 76
  Cancer 66
  Cardiomyopathies 138
  Cholesterol, High 100, 183–189
  Gallstones 43
  Gastritis 31
  Hypertension 129–130
  Hyperthyroidism 83
  Pancreatic disorders 41–42
  Panic disorders 89–90
  Pregnancy 15
  Proper daily diet & exercise 176, 192–193, 196–200, 206, 207, 208
  Ulcer 34
Doctor, Choice of 152–153

EKG 4, 74, 108
Emergencies 5, 7, 106
  Preparing for 154–167

Emergency Room visits 4, 5, 6
  Researching nearest 156
  How to handle 165–167
  Relatives accompanying 167
Emotions,
  High-impact-low-benefit 36, 76, 85–94, 100, 102, 110–111, 117, 140, 166, 170–171, 174, 179–182, 201
Emphysema 50, 104
Environmental illnesses 61–62, 64, 102
EPA 185–187
  Capsules 197–198
Esophagus, Disorders 12–28
  Achalasia 26, 27
  Diagnosis 28
  Erosion 18–19
  Infections 27
  Motility disorders 24–25
  Non-effective spasms 25, 86
  Nutcracker syndrome 25
  Rupture 22–23
  Tumors 27
  Ulcerated 23–24
Exercise 77, 101, 113, 129, 170–171, 174–182, 192–193, 195, 207
  Walking program 174–180

Faith, Need for 160, 164
Fat consumption 36, 43, 169, 184–185, 191, 193, 207
Fear, Dealing with 159–160
Fiber 187–188
Fibromyositis 75, 80

Gallbladder 43–45
Gas, Excess 19, 21
  Prevention of 21
Gastritis 29–32
  Causes 29–31
  Treatment 31–32

INDEX 223

Heart, Description of 97–98
Heart attack 1, 7, 108, 140–147
  Causes 140
  Death from 144–145
  Diagnosis 143–144
  Pain patterms 142
  Prevention 84
  Silent 143
  Treatment 145–147
  Survival 2, 3, 5
Hiatal hernia 14
Hypertension 69, 84, 128–129, 200, 201
  Therapy for 130
  See also *Diet,* Modifying your
Hyperthyroidism 82–83, 104
Hyperventilation 89, 90

Idiopathic disorders 63–64
Ileitis 63
Immune-suppressed patients 27, 55, 57, 73, 86
Inner voice work 182–183
Insurance, Medical 158–159
Intercostal neuritis 72–74

Klebsiella pneumonia 52, 56

Laughter, Therapeutic 94, 160, 161, 208
Left ventricle hypertrophy 128–130
Life-style changes 17, 94, 107, 110, 111, 113, 116, 129–130, 141, 168–209
Love, Need for (Vitamin L) 177, 195, 201, 202, 207, 209
Lungs 46–66. *See also* Pulmonary entries
Lupus 75. 119, 122

Mediastinum 67–71
Medications
  Acyclovir 57
  Alprazolam 90
  Amantadine 58

Aspirin 33, 103, 145.
Bentyl 16
Beta blockers 63, 90, 110–111, 117
Bethanecol 25
Calcium channel blockers 24, 26, 111, 117, 129
Captopril 111, 129
Carafate 34
Chenodeoxycholic acid 44
Chlorpromamide 63
Clonidine 84
Corgard 111
Cortisone 41, 72, 80, 123, 138
Coumadin 49, 50
Digitalis 117, 129
Dilantin 119
Diltiazem 111
Dipryridamole 49
Diuretics 41
Doxycycline 124
Erythromycin 57
Heparin 50
Hydrolazine 111, 119
Ibuprofen group 30
Imipramine 90
Inderal 111
Lopressor 111
Nifedipine 11
Nitroglygerin 24, 106, 108–110, 142–143
Penicillin 57, 124
Pepcid 16, 24
Procaine 119
Propanalol 117
Prostaglandin 32, 34
Quinidine 117
Reglan 21
Tagamet 16, 34
Tenormin 111
Tolbutamide 63
Ursodeoxycholic acid 44
Valium 89
Vancomycin 57

Verapamil 111, 138
Zantac 16, 34
Menetriere's disease
Mycoplasma 56
Myocardial infarction. *See* Heart attack
Myocarditis 122–124, 126
Myositis 78

Obesity 44, 47, 191–192
Osteoporosis 77
Oxygen, Home emergency use 156–157

Pacemaker 115–116, 118
Pain tolerance 32
Painkillers, Avoidance of 17
Pancreas, Disorders of 40–42
Panic disorder 87–91
　Emotional causes 88–89, 102
　Pain patterns 88, 102
　Physical causes 89–90, 190
　Treatment 90–91
Paramedics
　Calling 6, 7, 144, 155, 158
　Information for 161–165
Parathyroid gland disease 39
Perfectionism, Effects of 175, 192, 207
Pericardial effusion 41
Pericarditis 75, 117, 119–121, 147
Pets, Danger of infection from 54
Pheochromocytoma 104–105
Plaque 69, 100–101, 103, 109, 140, 190
Pleurisy 58–60
Pneumonia 55–58
Pneumothorax 60–61
Posture, Effects of poor 81
Pregnancy 15, 44, 103
Pseudomonas 56
Psychological causes for pain 85–94

Psychotherapy 153
Pulmonary emboli 7, 47–50
　Pain patterns 48
　Prevention 49
　Treatment 49–50
Pulmonary hypertension 50–51, 104
Purkinje fibers 104, 115

Reflux esophagitis 13–15, 98
Relatives of cardiovascular patients, Advice for 204–206, 209
Relaxation. *See* Stress, Reduction
Rheumatoid arthritis 63, 75, 119, 122
Rib, Fractured 7, 77–78

Sarcoid 68
Self-esteem 171, 181–182, 194
Sepsis 53
Serotonin 92
Sex 179
Sickle-cell anemia 81–82
Silent ischemia 141
Sinus node 115
Sodium 200, 208. *See also* Diet
Sphincter muscles 13–14, 19–26
　Disorders, Life-threatening 19–22
Spondylitis 75
Staphyloccocus 56
Sternum 67, 72, 74
Streptoccocus 54, 56
Stress 5, 58, 76, 80, 94, 141, 208
　Reduction 151–167, 176, 195
　Relaxation techniques 152–154, 159–160, 164, 167, 171
　Result of disease 30. *See also* Emotions, High-impact, etc.

Syphilis, Complications of 69, 70, 98, 122, 123, 124, 126–127. *See also* Syphilitic heart disease
Syphilitic heart disease 125–127

Thoracic spine disease 71
Thrombolysis 49
Thymus gland 67
Tuberculosis 52, 60
Tumors, Cardia 139
Type A personality 93–94, 152, 156
  Coronary risk for 94
  Treatment 94

Ulcers, Stomach 32–37, 38
  Causes 33
  Diagnosis 34, 38
  Treatment 34–37

Valley fever 52
Valve disorders 98, 131–135
  Dental involvement 133
Vascular system 97
Viruses 57, 72, 76, 122, 133, 136, 137
Visualization 66
Vitamins 58, 66, 77, 110, 116,
  Recommended 195–202

Water, Proper intake of 193–194, 208
Weight, Normal 191

Xiphodynia 78

Zollinger-Ellison syndrome 38–39